Free Fall

A MEMOIR

Free Fall

FELICITY JEAN

Note:

Some names and identifying details have been changed to protect the privacy of individuals. In order to maintain their anonymity in some instances I have changed the names of places, I may have changed some identifying characteristics and details such as physical properties, occupations and places of residence.

www. FelicityJeanAuthor.com

Author photograph by: Mariano Friginal
Book and Front Cover Design Concepts: GarReynaDesign.com
Editing by: C.J. Collins

ISBN #978-1-7345584-5-6 (ebook)
ISBN #978-1-7345584-8-7 (pbk)

Copyright © 2020 by Felicity Jean

All rights reserved. No part of this publication may be reproduced or transmitted in any form or by any means electronic or mechanical, including photocopy, recording, or any information storage and retrieval system, without permission in writing from both the copyright owner and the publisher.

DEDICATION

To my late husband,
who gave me messages
along the way.

Contents

	Prologue - Death Sentence	1
	SECTION 1 - MARK & JEAN	
Chapter 1	Closet [2011]	3
Chapter 2	Meeting [1997]	9
Chapter 3	Serendipity [1997 - 1998]	19
Chapter 4	Mom [1998]	29
Chapter 5	Destiny [1999 - 2000]	39
	SECTION 2 - DOCTORS & MEMORY LOSS	
Chapter 6	Signs & First Visit [2005]	45
Chapter 7	Second Opinion [2006]	57
Chapter 8	Hospice Trial Run [2008]	65
Chapter 9	Waiting Rooms [2008]	71
Chapter 10	Garden Talk [2009]	79
Chapter 11	Family Involvement [2010]	83
Chapter 12	Hallway [2010]	93
Chapter 13	Dad [2010]	103
Chapter 14	Realization [2010]	111
Chapter 15	Wellness Clinic Exit [2010]	115
Chapter 16	Hallucinations [2011]	125
Chapter 17	Family Notifications [2011]	131
Chapter 18	Movie Transition [APRIL 2012]	137
	SECTION 3 - HOSPITAL & ASSISTED LIVING	
Chapter 19	Embedded [MAY - JUNE 2012]	151
Chapter 20	Prey [JUNE - JULY 2012]	157
Chapter 21	Revealing Moments [JULY 2012]	169

Chapter	22	4th Trip to Hospital [JULY 2012]	181
Chapter	23	Angel Discharge Nurse [JULY 2012]	193
		SECTION 4 - HOSPICE CARE AT HOME	
Chapter	24	Hospice Care [JULY 2012]	199
Chapter	25	Decisions [AUGUST 2012]	211
Chapter	26	Release [AUGUST 2012]	219
		SECTION 5 - AFTER	
Chapter	27	Division [AUGUST 2012]	227
Chapter	28	Las Vegas [OCTOBER 2012]	231
Chapter	29	Transparent Touches [2012 - 2013]	237
Chapter	30	Messages [JULY - SEPTEMBER 2018]	243
		Epilogue	249
		References	251
		Acknowledgments	253
		About the Author	255

Prologue: Death Sentence

After our first date in the fall of 1997, Mark walked me to the front door of my home. The two-bedroom ranch house in Fresno was my first purchase after my divorce. It had taken me months to save up for the down payment. And finally, once it was mine, to me, it was a sanctuary. But it was time to take a new friend inside of it. I wondered if I should invite him in for a drink or if it seemed too forward. It only took me a nano-second to decide.

We sat on what was once my re-upholstered seventy's orange and green Polynesian sofa. It was now a clean, white, nubby-cloth contemporary, with wicker sides. A new couch for a new start, much like me trying to reinvent my single life.

I met handsome and tall Mark on a blind date. His preppy appearance, friendly conversation, warm demeanor, and lingering laughter grabbed my attention. I had waited 14 years, and was not eager to jump into anything serious, but, this new friendship seemed to fit. Was I ready for a commitment? Was he the right man?

Fast forward to 2000, and we were married. Six years later, in 2006, Mark was diagnosed with Early Onset Dementia, the kind that turned to Alzheimer's. Six years later in 2012, he passed away.

This is my story. How we at first thrived in our second marriage like two young lovebirds who had finally found each other. In Mark's declining years, as a spousal caregiver, I dealt with my husband's illness, our separate assets, and accepted, without doubt, gifts given to me by Mark, before, during, and after he passed from this world. I believe our love is a force of the heart that will endure forever, and I think with true conviction, that Mark's spirit has contacted me over and over, sending me his devotion from the other side.

SECTION 1 - MARK & JEAN

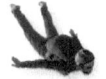

Chapter 1: Closet
[2011]

It was summer of 2011, and I was fixing tea in the kitchen of our home and heard the loud rustle of newspapers in the background. I walked into the living room and saw Mark's face, the muscles on his cheeks contracting, lips pressed, while he complained his lip balm disappeared.

"Lip balm?" I asked stupidly.

"Yes," he demanded. "Where is it?"

I thought he was settled and watching the football game while I finished in the kitchen. He said, "I think the cleaning lady stole my things. They're not in my top drawer."

"Mark, I don't think…"

"Yes, stealing from us."

"…anybody is stealing your…things." I took a deep breath and decided to flow with his outburst rather than correct him. "Let me see if I can find them."

Not happy with his tirade and frankly so fatigued, I'd almost dropped a teacup in the kitchen sink and broke it. My fingers were claws I pressed into my jeans so he wouldn't see them. Spending what little free time I had, digging for items he misplaced or lost, a waste of time and nothing I could afford to deal with. Who else will do it?

I swallowed and forced myself to remember his internal terrorist. The disease completely took over his brain. Tears pricked my eyes. More and more each month, it seemed I struggled through an invisible fog to get anything accomplished. Today was no exception.

Fog or no fog strung out or angry as a hornet at his constant obsession with small items he'd thrown out, like a kid with a used stick of gum or left in the garden by accident. I had to do this. I had to help.

He pestered me with false needs and concerns, "I'm out of lip balm. I'm out of nasal spray. Where are my sunglasses? Have you seen them?"

"I haven't seen them, Mark."

"I wore them yesterday."

"I don't think so."

"When we went to the grocery store."

"That was a week ago."

"No, it wasn't."

The barrage never stopped.

I repeatedly purchased more, at least three times in the last few weeks. Frustrated, I hastily walked to the bedroom and looked in the four dresser drawers and tore everything upside down to find his missing things with no luck. I went to his closet and looked in the pockets of all his button-down plaid shirts, Dockers and jackets, nothing there. I looked up high, where I placed his shiny dress shoes, but couldn't reach high without a step ladder. I previously moved his good leather shoes up to that shelf to clean his closet to organize and simplify things, as per doctor's orders.

Because I couldn't reach, I went into the garage and located the step ladder. We remodeled the bedroom flooring with uneven and bumpy, large slate tiles. Carefully, I made sure I was balanced and on level ground. My heart raced, beads of sweat surfaced above my upper lip, along with hot sweaty armpits, while I stood on the highest step. I looked in his closet and searched through his dress shoes stored on the upper shelf. As I pulled the shoes down, I found his things.

I took a deep breath and yelled, "Mark, please come in here."

When he came in, I ignored him, afraid of my anger, rummaging in the shoes.

After a few seconds, I turned and looked at him. His expression was one I never saw on him before. He was stern and agitated red in the face.

While on the ladder, I waved my hands and yelled, "Here are the things you thought were stolen. You hid them! Here's your nasal spray, your lip balm, and your sunglasses!"

When I stepped off the ladder, he grabbed one of my arms hard, hit my other arm and threw me on the bed. The internal terrorist completely took over his decision making. This man who physically assaulted me was not my husband.

SECTION 1 - MARK & JEAN

I wept hysterically, shook with fear and immediately called my brother-in-law, Robert, but couldn't reach him. Then I called my daughter. "Ann, please come over. Mark and I argued and he hit me. I need you."

"Oh no! Mom, I'll come right over."

* * *

It was just a year earlier I looked all over the house for Mark, (when the disease was in the early stages) and found him sitting in the kitchen at the nook, snacking on Jamocha almond fudge ice cream right out of the carton, holding a wet soiled dish towel around it, eating it with a big smile, after I caught him. He looked out into the yard we called our forest, "Carmel Cozy." He fell in love with the large, twenty-year-old pine trees when he first saw the house. It reminded him of the mountains.

From the kitchen windows, you saw a beautiful view of the pine trees with Capella squirrels chirping on branches and baby tears and Begonia flowers blooming out of the ceramic pots. You walked out the sliding glass doors to our wooden deck and sat at two glass-top tables with umbrellas covering them. In the winter you were heated by a tall stainless-steel lamp and heater.

I enjoyed our cute, black and white King Charles Cavalier puppy, Barni, short for Barnabas, running around. His long ears almost touched the ground at the bottom of his stubby clumsy legs. Mark's daughter, Tammy, suggested we get the puppy. She had one and thought the dog would be company for her dad.

The neighbors never complained when we hosted parties with family and friends gathered in our backyard. I left the sliding doors open from the kitchen and great room and often you heard loud stereo music playing along with conversation and everyone's laughter.

The Mark I married ate right, worked out daily, and paid attention to detail. He was the most easygoing and even-tempered person I ever met. It was hard to confront him about his doctor ordered diet.

I sat across from him at our table for two and smelled the irresistible chocolate and coffee-flavored ice cream saturating the dish towel, dripping with the chocolate all over on his hands and arms. He handed me a

SECTION 1 - MARK & JEAN

spoonful and I accepted the heaping portion he placed in my mouth slightly dripping from the side of my lips.

I remember it was a good day. He smiled and looked at me with love in his heart. Fast forward a year later, not only had I rehomed my sweet dog, I no longer lived in our home with my husband. I didn't know who Mark was anymore.

* * *

While Ann stayed to help keep Mark company (he didn't remember what just happened, grabbing or throwing me), I called and left a message for the doctor from the Neurology group at the UCSF office in Fresno to inform her Mark hit me. I was lucky to have such a great daughter, and Mark especially loved her. She could keep him calm with her sweet disposition.

The doctor called back. I asked if Mark needed different meds to help with the changes in his behavior. She cautioned me again to lock up his meds and anything dangerous. She also told me never to challenge a person with the illness my husband had. They become combative, lashing out, striking out, hitting and beating.

She said, "Do not take this lightly. It will happen again."

Things had to be safe. I already purchased a lockbox to gather all the meds and dangerous things, but never locked everything away. I began to do this while Ann kept him occupied. He sat with her on the sofa, as if nothing happened. They chatted freely. He quickly seemed to forget.

I walked into the garage for the lock box and placed it on top of the dryer in the laundry room and quickly picked up handfuls of his medications, scissors, pocket knives in his drawer, clippers, alcohol, letter openers and secured them.

Completely exhausted, shaky, and emotional, I tossed and turned in bed later, and began to think things over. I could no longer be in denial: this was real, I could no longer travel with the speed of traffic, like a normal person or couple. More in order was, "Caution: Children at Play." I learned the rules and stuck to them. Slow down. Keep us safe.

I wanted to think of good things. I reminisced of when we met, through my friend Conn. I dated Conn previously and was glad he remained my friend for years, or I might not have met Mark. Conn, never the marrying kind, but being my good friend, never forgot my constant mantra, I can't seem to meet an available good man. You know what I like, why don't you find someone for me? Please be on the lookout for somebody nice with a great sense of humor.

SECTION 1 - MARK & JEAN

SECTION 1 - MARK & JEAN

Chapter 2: Meeting
[1997]

Soon after I met Mark in 1997, I was ready to start a new relationship. Thus, I accepted his invitation to take a jump into unchartered space in a skydive. My idea, but after I thought about it, I breathed faster and my hands shook.

My mouth watered and my heart pounded out of my chest that morning on the way to his place. I parked my car in front of his condo. He stepped out to greet me, "Good morning sunshine, come in."

His condo was a well-kept, modest place with space enough for a single person. He gave me a quick tour before we left. Not to stereotype, but it was a typical after-divorce kind of place. His furniture was neatly tucked in tight, like overcrowded people at church on Easter Sunday. He loved the outdoors and the thing that struck me was the small patio. I said to myself like a blushing college girl, He won't live in this condo for very long!

On the drive to the Madera airport, a sunrise illuminated the sky with layers of golden lines over the crimson and purple skies to underscore the dark Sierra Nevada Mountains at the start of a beautiful clear morning. Reflections of polished highlights hovered over the worn metal building, as our trophy day began upon entering this adventure.

In the airplane hangar, we released our instructors of any possible liability should things go wrong in the adventure of gliding like a bird.

Our instructor, about six feet tall with blond curly hair and freckles, greeted us with a warm smile. The short jovial videographer looked like a cute Christmas elf. He introduced himself and asked, "Are you in for a great experience?"

I pulled my hair behind my ears. "Great! I want an adventure. How long is the ride?"

"We'll go over all that."

Mark's brother Robert surprised us to support and rally. They didn't look like brothers, Mark tall and thin, and his brother shorter and more buff. After their jokes and jabs back and forth, you could tell without a doubt they were related.

The instructor handed us all the paperwork and wanted some vitals for our jumpsuits.

"How tall are you?" he asked me.

"I'm five-three."

Mark came back, "I'm six-two."

I took a deep breath and had faith all would be well. About then, they brought in Mark's overalls and said with a slight snicker, "Hope these are long enough for you." I watched while Mark stepped into them and zipped them up. Yep, they fit. Other than grabbing his cojones, they worked. I'm sure he had a major wedgie.

Then Mark said, "I'll be right back."

He returned wearing a baseball cap with an attached long ponytail hanging from the back, a mischievous twinkle in his eyes and his signature infectious laughter. I knew from that moment that he was my soulmate.

He's mine, I thought. He's so beautiful and funny!

We went over the safety list, but more importantly, we were hooked together with our instructor partner. Our ride was fifteen minutes long before drop off, at a descent of 120 miles per hour, with a free fall at forty-five to sixty-seconds. We jumped tandem and somersaulted with our instructor individually while being videotaped by the experienced jumper elf.

Excited, I offered to go first. The instructor and I walked to the runway out to the plane, and I climbed in on two steps through the opening of the missing door. The infamous opening revealed the authenticity of our bravery. The videographer offered his hand and held my hand to help me onto the resting airplane. Right about then, my mouth started watering. Where did this come from? I'd been looking forward to it. I bit the inside of my cheeks.

The gutted cockpit held one seat and the pilot already seated, looked our way and smiled.

SECTION 1 - MARK & JEAN

"Jean, sit parallel on the floor next to the pilot in the opposite direction. Face toward the back of the plane." My instructor said.

"OK," I was up for it, yet more nervous than ever.

I looked and smelled the old and rusty sides and the back of the pilot's worn leather seat. I felt like I was accepted into the fraternity. No turning back. My instructor tapped me on the shoulders and asked me to scoot up. He told me to sit between his legs, right in front of him. That way, he could strap me securely to him when we reached eight thousand-foot elevation. Up close and personal, I just met this guy. There was enough room for me, the pilot, my instructor, who was more like my conjoined twin, and the videographer who sat across from us.

I heard the propeller turning. My head exploded with excitement. Then the engine started rumbling, like an animal coaching its offspring. I barely heard when the instructor yelled, "Everybody ready?

"Yes," We all sang in unison.

Airborne, we ascended. I looked out and saw the lay of the land sectioned off with green vegetation of farmland, brown parcels with rows of agriculture, a lush green golf course and bluff hill homes on the edge of the San Joaquin River.

As he secured my straps and shook me back into reality, my heart began to race. My upper body pulsed heat to my neck and cheeks. My instructor scooted us to the edge of the open door and turned our bodies to face the sky. He pulled my forehead close to his body, while he held his left hand to the side closest to the front of the plane. Positioned in front of him, the cold wind blew fiercely at my face, my cheeks pulsated at high speed, like batter flying off the side of a bowl. My Staccato right then was, You can do it, you can do it! At this point, I don't recall my legs dangling off the bottom of the plane, as if they morphed into my winged brain telling me to breathe, but instead, I think I stopped breathing. My other senses took over, while my ears heard the loud music mix of the vibration of the wind song.

"Ready to somersault?" said my instructor.

"YESSSS!" I replied.

SECTION 1 - MARK & JEAN

And heads out first, away we rolled. In the middle of clouds up 10,000 feet. Temperatures both cool and warm brushed my face. We flew horizontally with our arms and hands stretched out, and we waved them against the blowing forceful wind; I had wings like a bird floating in the air how it felt in my dreams. I looked in front and side to side. I saw a fantasy land of clouds, like large pieces of white cotton candy with the backdrop of blue skies. The toggles pulled, I felt a jolt to position us vertically, as flickers of light and the reflection of the large parachute canopy opened. We headed closer to the ground in a few seconds or minutes. I can't remember moving my hands, but my body jerked, as my tandem partner maneuvered the toggles to help us land on the right target.

It was an unmatched, heavenly adventure for Mark and me.

Mark's brother, Robert, proudly smiled and laughed, as he welcomed us in, and photographed for evidence our jump! We landed steady with both feet down, no falling to the ground. We both gave high fives to one another. Mark's smile, infectious laughter, humor and fun we shared, stamped my heart - Forever.

At the same time a part of me still skeptical, remained cautious of the future. Was I trying to build a barrier so I wouldn't get hurt? He seemed nice and fun. I had so many questions still unanswered. Was he on his best behavior, would it change later? Would he be there for me emotionally in time? I'd been single too long. I needed to take a deep breath, slow down and go with it.

* * *

On the way to hike in Yosemite, Mark drove through foothills in a rolling hills community and stopped to introduce me to his good friends, Betty and Sonny, who lived on the way. Blond-haired, blue-eyed Betty opened the front door and smiled with her great spirit of personality, hospitality, and fun, like that of my mother, a deja-vu. But, Mom had black-hair and brown-eyes.

SECTION 1 - MARK & JEAN

Back in the SUV almost to Yosemite, Mark pulled to the side to park along the way and took pictures, but first asked, "How's this for some pictures?"

"Great!" I shouted, fluffed up my hair. Back to being the blushing college girl, nervous, excited, I fumbled for my lipstick, pulled the visor down. Then realized. What was I doing? We were in the mountains. Relax.

He got out of the SUV, opened the back and started going through the Nikon camera and tripod equipment. I stood in the back and watched him find the angle for the right spot.

"You know, morning and late afternoon are the best times to get the best shots. Even when there's an overcast. Drama in the sky, always a good time." As he moved this way and that, he turned his baseball hat around with the bill in the back. I snuck a few of him with my little Canon camera, while he took pictures. His knees bent and squatted low. I tried to ignore the tickle of hair blown on my face from the cool breeze. I just wanted a good one of him while he took his shots.

No matter what the season, Mark's photography captured God's creation of nature's beautiful trees, monolith rock formations, waterfalls, creeks, and habitat for deer, birds, and bears. The rich sounds of the waterfalls overwhelmed me with gratitude and fed my spirit.

It became my desire to keep this relationship maintained for years, and to see these mountains from a different view each time. This casual, active, activity I craved and didn't know it until I tasted it. So sick of dates with the same dinner and drinks, I no longer wanted to be wined and dined. I needed to breathe and take in the freshness of nature all around us. It had been a long time since I'd felt loved by a man.

Back in the car, he found a perfect place for our picnic, near a meadow and surrounded by towering cedar and pine trees. He took wine, a chardonnay, and a merlot, Gouda cheese, and apples cut into wedges.

We looked along the face of the mountain rock wall and watched rock climbers with Mark's binoculars. The warmth of his company; and God's sun embraced us both, while he spoke openly of his former marriage and the good that came out of it, his daughters.

"Has your divorce tainted your belief in marriage?" I asked hesitantly.

"No, I believe in marriage, but I don't feel like I need another one right now. I would like a good relationship someday, just not now." In a moment of pause, I couldn't help but think, What's that supposed to mean? Am I wasting my time? Are we in different time zones? Give it time.

Was I silly? – Trying too much to predict our future together already? As badly as his first marriage hurt him, I had battle scars with my first one. This marriage would be the second for both of us. Heat flamed my face. What marriage? What was I doing?

On the way home, I watched the scenery while we talked about our lives. Even though previously, I was taken aback by his comments, the ease of our conversations demonstrated the closeness we had already developed. While he drove, I looked at him and reminisced of the day, the times I stood near him. Watched him take pictures, I loved the way he dressed, his red plaid shirt, suede tan vest, skinny jeans, and leather hiking boots. How he wore his baseball hat, how he smelled woodsy and talked to me like I was someone important and interesting. Attracted to him, I wanted to get closer. Until he leaned toward me, looked my way, and said, "I'm ready whenever you are." He sounded serious. He looked straight ahead at the road at a car passing us.

I imagine he took in the day and hoped never let go of those feelings, and also looked forward to the day he could get closer. I was ready to get close but thought it too soon. I looked at him and laughed, didn't know how to respond, and thought, So sweet, tender, and gentle. I loved him for the grace and respect he gave me.

He had a great voice and loved to sing along to the music and often said, "Take it." I can't remember what he sang that day, but I wouldn't put it past him to sing along to the Bee Gees' song, You Should Be Dancing, except he would have changed it to, You Should Be Singing! I had a scratchy voice, couldn't carry a tune, and shy about singing along, so he sang to me.

"Do you have plans for the next few years?" I asked.

"I'd like to travel more. I'll probably work a few more years." He kept his eyes on the road. I looked at his slender profile with a smooth fair complexion and aviator sunglasses.

SECTION 1 - MARK & JEAN

"Do you think you'll ever marry again?" There, I asked it.

"I don't know. The divorce was pretty nasty." He did not want to marry again. He was so much fun that day, but his conversation disclosed some unavailability for commitment. It made me sad.

One evening, he invited me to a charity event with headliner Jack Jones, which included dinner, dancing, and entertainment in a decorated airplane hangar. The night didn't end there, as a tip from his barber lured us to a blues club called, Not Your Mama's. Even though we dressed for the charity event, and underdressed upon entering the blues club, this place was already almost standing room only, with well-dressed couples in suits, hats, and shiny shoes, and they knew how to shake their booties.

The party of four, Mark, me, Sonny, and Betty, were minorities in our attire; but determined not to feel intimidated for our lack of dress and dancing ability. We squatted into the last booth left and meant for us, and tried to act somewhat incognito to blend in. Even if none of us danced, the music and crowd entertained us. We walked in as a group of two couples, but that didn't stop a stranger who asked me to dance. I politely said, "No, thank you, not right now."

"It wasn't polite to say no." New best girlfriend, Betty, silently whispered in my ear.

"Then, we're going together," I whispered back to her.

"My friend would love to dance. We'll both come." I turned and replied to the gentleman.

The empty dance floor reserved for its three new dancers, me, Betty, and smooth-dancing African American gentleman. No one else came to the dance floor! Both Betty and I danced, not doing our best expression of dance under the spotlights, for fear we didn't measure up to the standards of this club, and worse - the fear of being asked to dance again. We moved slowly with stiff shoulders hardly moving around and tried to look dull, almost like penguins, with only our feet moving.

Afterward, Betty, Mark, Sonny, and I all entered the dance floor. Mark, with his hands up high, moving all around. Betty whispered her advice to me, "Tell Mark to stop dancing that way. The crowd thinks he's making fun of them."

SECTION 1 - MARK & JEAN

That night, everyone's expression of dance was never forgotten by their significant others for years, especially by Mark. He later held his arms stiffly down on his side, mocking the way Betty and I had done, and said, "Is this all you got?"

We sat at his patio many evenings in deep conversation, while he calmly told a compelling story, then slipped in a one-line zinger and took me by surprise. I snorted out my nose at some of his outlandish punch-lines, rubs, and jokes.

Sometimes he sketched a picture of a plant or tree to show me an example of something he wanted to see in his yard. I always thought he was a frustrated artist who wanted to work outdoors, sketching and painting landscapes and animals. Somehow, he ended up working indoors as a successful real estate professional who worked with numbers and analysis.

I trusted him, and we talked about anything to challenge each other with our voice of opinion. As Christians, we respected each other's background of religious teachings. I loved our time together and hoped there was more to come. My rational side told me I could cope with just being friends, but my raw emotional side was selfish and needed more. Oh yes, I could spend my time doing the things I wanted to do, read, take classes and write. In truth I wanted a partner to love and share my life with. I didn't blame him but didn't know if I could stay casual friends or even best friends. How shallow was I? My heart was torn. It ached when I was close to him when I was away from him, and it ached for us to belong to each other.

In spite of his commitment phobia, Mark and I started to develop a great friendship; we got to know our true self without the complication of getting physical too soon. We allowed layers of our internal shields to come off slowly. Months of deep conversations, dinner, drinks, and a bonding held both of us beyond our control. He fished, hunted, hiked, and traveled. I hiked and worked out, but was it enough to sustain me in a longer hiking trip? I wrote down my specific wish list, visualized it, and believed it. Mark had everything on my list.

No bones about it, was I an idiot? I would never force Mark to marry me. But I wanted him so badly. I wanted him more than I wanted anyone for a very long time. He was the man of my dreams who raised me high above the clouds.

But would he overcome his fear of marriage again? Not a patient person; I wanted to bean Mark on the head. How could he not see the obvious? And to get my mind off all uncertainty, I visualized in my silly head - Try to enjoy the moments - The right now - But could I? Or was I about to come crashing down?

* * *

SECTION 1 - MARK & JEAN

SECTION 1 - MARK & JEAN

Chapter 3: Serendipity
[1997 -1998]

Before meeting Mark, at forty-seven, I regressed, like a college kid coming home after failing her finals. I moved in with my parents. I had previously rented my house in Fresno, California, and accepted another job in commercial real estate sales in Los Angeles. Due to the downfall of the economy in the late '80s and '90s, humbled, I filed for bankruptcy. My parents were great. No job. No man. No life. No home runs...I think back to my introduction to Mark in 1997...

I received a call from my good friend, Conn. "Jean, I met a great guy. I think you should call him. He's the marrying kind. I think he'd be good to you." Sounds like Conn has a man-crush.

"What does he look like?" I asked. Pushing fifty years old, my stomach flipped. I jumped up and looked in the mirror for wrinkles on my face. Seated on the bed in the same childhood bedroom that I grew up in, I hadn't been on a date for a few years.

"He wears glasses. Has a receding hairline. Tall and good-looking. The best part, an attention-getting laugh. He talked about his nasty divorce. He said," 'It's difficult to meet a good woman.' "I told Mark," 'I know the person for you. She's easy on the eyes.' "Jean, I have his number."

"I'm not calling him. I trust you, give him my number. Hey, what about his laugh? Is it annoying or what's noticeable?" I asked.

"It's spontaneous. Like someone is tickling him. Stops for a breather and then starts again," Conn said. Quick to phone me that next morning, Conn said Mark was cordial, knowledgeable of the outdoors, hunting and fishing, and funny.

They met at his place during the annual dove hunting season. Conn, well known in the community for his philanthropy, optimistic personality, and zest for life, told great stories and known for his Conn-isms. I had been to his ranch north of Fresno in Madera. I thought about the ranch, electric in the mornings with sunlight weaved through the oak trees that flickered diamonds on the river. At the end of that day, the guests including

SECTION 1 - MARK & JEAN

Mark, enjoyed the views of the landscape and river. They celebrated the day's festivities with drinks and dinner at the home's large wooden deck.

* * *

My only other blind date with my ex-husband, was when he was twenty and I, seventeen. We married six months later. We divorced after seventeen years, and I was alone for seventeen years, enough penance for sure. Don't get me wrong. I wouldn't change my decision to marry that young. At the time I was seventeen going on thirty-five. No one believed we planned to have a baby, but we did. Blessed to have my daughter Ann. Born a premie at three pounds, two and a half ounces, she grew into a 5' 4" adult with brown hair and eyes, and full of wisdom. Anytime I asked for advice, I trusted her direction. She knew what path to take like a river knows a path and where to meander.

* * *

After Conn called, I sat on the bed of my childhood bedroom. The mattress squeaked on springs. The fourteen-year-old of my youth looked at the original furniture, white antique dresser, matching side tables with gold knobs, and in my head, screamed, "Yikes! What the hell are you doing?" Disorientation. Falling through space. I should have been used to it. I wasn't. Until the best part of this room hit me. Near the window, I smelled the fragrant buds, my mom's favorite roses. After my brother and I left home to go pursue our endeavors, she watered, pruned, and cared for them religiously, like she did for us when we were younger. My dad loved to fish and hunt. If my dad enjoys the outdoors and Mark does, maybe it's a good sign. My dad loves his family, is respectful of others, and respected.

I loved my parents, but I couldn't wait to get my house back from the renters. They showed their affection by being food pushers who filled my plate as if it was my last meal. My mom's specialty was home-made buttery mashed potatoes, fried chicken, corn on the cob, and al a mode boysenberry pie.

Still nervous. My heart raced. Sick to my stomach and clammy, in and out of the bathroom, it was like I was back in high school. I didn't leave the house, excited for this awaited phone call from Conn's friend, Mark. I slapped my forehead. What was I doing? Did I trust Conn enough to go through with this? Maybe I'll call Ann to get her opinion.

"Ann?"

"That's me," she said, using our usual banter. "What's up?"

"I'm about to barf."

"Oh, great. What happened?"

"A man is going to call me for a date."

"No, kidding? Do you remember how to date?"

"Ha, ha."

"What's he look like? A troll?"

"Funny. He's quite handsome I'm told."

"Well, you have nothing to worry about. You look great."

"Thanks. I needed that."

"I mean it, I love you, Mom."

"I know."

"This is going to be hard."

"I know."

That evening, my seventy-one-year old Mom walked into the bedroom like a sleek cat with a secret. She held the phone in her hand while she covered the mouthpiece and whispered to me, "It's a man for you." Her eyes were brown sparkles, and her smile, contagious and naughty. She threw the phone into my hands. I shook, I tripped on my foot, caught myself and looked at her. I imagine I wore a joker smile and a contorted forehead, like the smashed sock-faces in a jar. Then I snatched the phone from her. I pushed her out (her giggles escaping even as she hoofed it) and closed the door, and said, "Hello."

"Hi, I'm Mark, Conn's friend."

"Yes, so nice of you to call."

"I haven't done anything like this in a long time."

"Me either. Feels odd."

"Strange. Agreed. But I'd like to try if you want to try."

SECTION 1 - MARK & JEAN

Our conversation lasted for hours. It was a consensual night, a feeding frenzy of exchange on common subjects, which did end with an invitation to dinner in two days. I looked forward to meeting him, but it wouldn't be easy. Even though I was single for a few years, to walk into a bar alone wasn't easy. At least the restaurant in Fresno he chose was dimly lit, subdued, with many booths, lots of elbow room, and our conversation somewhat private, meeting time of 6:30 p.m. on Wednesday with an older crowd was perfect.

Getting ready that night, I said, "Mom, I'm tired of trying to look cute or sexy for men. I don't think I'll wear makeup tonight."

Mom was old-school and wasn't having it. I remember how she looked. Her lips tightly closed while she refrained from laughter, and her hands on her hips. "What? Are you kidding? You look like a sock puppet without makeup. I wouldn't risk it! No one wants to date a sock puppet." She said.

Not taking any chances (Who wanted a pale-faced sock puppet?), I wore the dreaded makeup. I tried on several outfits, all thrown on the bed, standing on a chair and looked in the mirror. I decided on a special navy-blue sleeveless, silk blouse with a small print matching skirt for this blind date, one that made me look skinnier. I also wore two-inch sandals to make my 5' 3" look taller.

Conn did a good sales job with the impression he gave me. I had to use my "A" game. Going into this evening, I had the background, but I wanted to see the other side of him. Was Mark family-oriented and faithful to God?

Fifteen minutes late, I snuck into the restaurant's bathroom for one last look to make sure my lips, makeup, hair looked good, and boobs were in the proper place. Mom always said, 'a come and get me look was necessary.' Maybe a little cleavage wouldn't hurt.

Still, my mind shouted at me: WHAT ARE YOU DOING, JEAN?!

"Go away," I said to my mind. "Just go away."

I sucked in a deep breath, which sounded desperate and pistol-whipped as I wiped raspberry-colored lipstick off my front teeth. Well, too bad. Free fall, I thought. Here I go.

SECTION 1 - MARK & JEAN

I hoped Mark was in the restaurant. Waiting for me. I walked in, and he was in a corner booth, looking good, as Conn described. He stood up and greeted me with a light and friendly hug, and we both sat. I said, "Sorry, I'm late, but I wanted to make sure you got here first."

"No problem, glad you're here."

While I sat, I noticed photographs on the table but said nothing. Dressed preppy with a button-down plaid, cotton shirt, khaki pants, and loafers, Mark was tall, thin-framed, and had green eyes. Age had blown away some of his gray hair, a swimmer's hairline look-a-like. Oh well, here we are. At least the shimmer of gold dust in his eyes overcompensates for his lack of hair.

A little self-conscious, I looked to see if I knew anyone. No one was sitting at the U-shaped bar, nor at the immediate booths. Relieved. I looked at the photographs on the table and ready to pick them up, but he beat me to it. He picked up his college picture first, a full head of hair, 40 years younger, which made me smile. He showed me a picture of his two adult daughters.

"Great pictures of you and your daughters. They look like beauty queens." I heard from Conn their mom was blond and cunning. I wonder what she looks like? Maybe, he doesn't like brunettes.

"Thanks. They are my girls." He beamed.

"Do they live in Fresno?"

"No, they live five hours away." His eyes twinkled as he talked about them.

"You must miss them that far away." As I handed him the photos back, he brushed my fingers. Was that on purpose?

"I do. I drive to see them occasionally." He smiled and looked at me.

"Are you still working?" I asked.

"Yes, I'm in the financial world."

"I'm in real estate. Previously, in banking," I said. He stared at me. It seemed long. This is nice for a change. He's making me melt, and my face is getting hot. I wonder if he's comparing me to his ex-wife. Is he over the divorce? God, this is awful. My stomach is all fluttery.

Knowledgeable on a variety of subjects, I soon realized that Conn was right in his assessment of him, quick-witted and a laugh that lingered, a magnet that pulled the laughter right out of me. Our conversation flowed easily, and I was at home with his warm demeanor. I wanted to see him again. Was I that easy? Or an idiot?

At the end of the evening, the one person I knew, the owner, dropped by our table to thank us. With a mischievous smile, he looked at me and said, "Please don't make him wait so long next time."

While Mark walked me to my car, he said, "I'll call again. If you want me to? Maybe we could meet again for dinner." I said yes while I unlocked my car. I turned to say thank you when he hugged me and gave me a quick peck. My inner voice went on overdrive. The timing seemed right. I dated younger and older men, but not the marrying kind of man. I wanted to give this possible relationship time. That is if he continued to pursue me. And if he was too slow, I might pursue him!

The next evening Mark invited me to dinner in two days. We met at a steakhouse/bar in a trendy area of town, called the Tower District, frequented by a younger crowd. This restaurant sat in the hub of a neighborhood known for its artistic and colorful people. The older commercial buildings and homes revitalized as a smaller version to mimic Sunset Boulevard in Los Angeles with galleries, artist studios, theatre, trendy fashions, and great restaurants. This happy-hour enjoyed a good following for the appetizers of delicious steak bites, potato skins, and pizzas. I especially liked to watch the stand-out retro women who wore vintage clothing of vibrant yellow and green paisley and tie-dyed prints, very pale makeup, thin eyebrows, and dark red lips.

I walked under the canopy entry into the restaurant, along a rail with a step down into the bar area. Mark sat and glanced back to see me walk in and stood. Noisy with conversations, laughter, and subtle music in the background, you heard the strumming of a guitar player. Mark leaned toward me with a hug and a cheek kiss. That moment my stomach leaped. I didn't want to spend the rest of my life alone. My inner voice-call intuition-trusted him and thought: He is a good man.

He asked me what I wanted to drink, and I ordered a Chardonnay. He raised his hand to the bartender and ordered my drink. Both family-oriented, social, worked in the real estate world and loved adventure. He had long relationships with his friends, saw his mother every week for lunch, and

SECTION 1 - MARK & JEAN

was close to his daughters. We both read, enjoyed gardening, and I fished with my dad. We also shared our differences. I didn't hunt, I was from a Hispanic family, and he was from an English/German family. In our discussions, our energy seemed equally matched.

"What would you like to do that you haven't done?" He asked.

"I've had dreams I fly. - A different kind of flying. - Swimming in the air, elevating myself up in the sky doing somersaults and I loved it. I want to jump out of an airplane." I really wanted to do it, but I wondered if he thought I was out of my mind, or tried to impress him.

"Let's go and do it!" He held and shook both my hands.

"I can't afford that."

"I can." I'll buy it for your birthday.

My impression of him and his age changed. He was young at heart and wanted to do fun and adventurous things. He was exciting and alluring to me in a different way and not a physical way. I didn't understand it, wouldn't question it, but I wanted to go on this magic ride as long as he kept inviting me.

I decided to tell my daughter, Ann. I cradled the phone in my childhood bedroom at the end of the hallway. My parents cooked dinner in the kitchen at the other end of the house. "Ann, it's Mom. I'm going on a very daring date."

"Wow. With Mark, the man you've been seeing?"

"Yes. And you won't believe what we're going to do?"

"It's too soon for a cruise."

I laughed. "No. Not that."

"A trip to Napa? You can't go without me. I want to taste the Pinot. I've heard the crops this year are amazing."

I laughed again. "No. That's not it."

She sighed. "I give up."

"Skydiving."

* * *

I thought about what Conn said about Mark. My other voice wondered why Mark's wife left him. How could anyone leave him? It was only a year since his divorce. I didn't know if he was capable or ready for another relationship. I'm not sure if the timing is right. Is he gone hunting and fishing too much? I wanted someone who wanted to spend time with me. But how much is too much time together, that he might lose interest? My mind drove me insane. Scared, excited, sick to my stomach, my body floated. Horrible trying to sort it. I didn't want to play games. I wanted this to flow easily. The one thing I did know for certain, I wanted to try. Trying was never easy for me. I thought of living in my parent's house at forty-eight years old. NO-NO-NO, I thought. Get on with it, girlfriend. Life was going by without my permission. I had to do something. Change. Get out there. Jump from the safe ledge of being alone.

* * *

In 1998, after returning from dinner out, Mark and I sat on my deck. A lovely evening with a gentle breeze moved the oak tree branches to fan us cool. The deck was designed around three large oak trees, carefully boxed in and preserved with square redwood benches. I smelled the fragrance of honeysuckle blossoms and roses in the air. I enjoyed this backyard deck in the first home I purchased as a single woman, with a sense of pride. However, I was more proud of him. He met almost all of the items on my list: family oriented, Christian, loving, and fun.

"Thanks, Jean, this is such a great evening. I love spending time with you." He looked at me with a smile, leaned over and kissed me. Be patient, don't say anything yet.

"I love this house and the backyard. But I don't feel safe. I want something in a gated community." I had to discuss my desire for a long term commitment. At other times, he seemed unavailable to commit to our relationship. I went inside to get us an after-dinner drink of wine. I hoped this night would be our time to talk about it.

"Well, what do you think I should do?" I asked.

"It might not be a bad idea to move. Have you looked anywhere?" He looked at me with his head tilted and his hands on his chin.

"I've looked a little, but not aggressively. I love this yard. But, I don't have time or the money for the maintenance of the landscape. The large tree trimming and cleaning are expensive."

"Why don't I come over tomorrow? I could help you with trimming some shrubs?"

"I appreciate it. But I'm thinking of future planning." I couldn't believe he didn't offer something for a long term solution.

"Mark, I would like to discuss our relationship. I need to know if you are planning to marry eventually. If not, I need to know. I don't want to invest time with no future." I kept my eyes on him.

"I can't commit to anything right now. My daughter is getting married in a few months. Her mother does not want to include you at the wedding. She's not taking anyone either. I've been separated for over a year. Almost legally divorced. My daughter is afraid her mother would cause a scene." He looked at me. Said he enjoyed my company but wasn't ready to commit.

A red flag, he had a controlling family. He was separated and almost legally divorced before I met him.

"This is unacceptable. I don't want to waste my time. Maybe you should leave." I waited. My face flushed red and heated down to my neck.

"Jean, maybe I should give you some time. Think it over. Let's sleep on this." He looked at me intently, as if he wanted me to change my mind. Then he got up, and I stood. I followed him to the door. I controlled my tears and composure until I walked him to the door. I went into my bedroom, lay on the bed, and started sobbing.

He wasn't ready. I moved on and left the relationship. Single for much longer, I understood where he was. Just the same, our relationship felt right. Devastated and sad, our timing was off.

A few months later, a friend made an introduction and I reluctantly dated someone else to fill the absence. Also, I focused on my work in banking and real estate.

SECTION 1 - MARK & JEAN

SECTION 1 - MARK & JEAN

Chapter 4: Mom
[1998]

I screamed and caught everyone's attention. My dad called at 3:00 p.m. in November 1998. His voice cracked when he told me the hospital notified him. My mother was hit by a car.

At my desk, I shook while I tried to compose myself. Customers stood in the teller line and turned to look at me. Voices in my head started: This is not good. Please help me God, call Ann. My gut told me it was bad. My supervisor asked what happened, then offered to drive me to the hospital right away. I took deep breaths and called Ann. "Grandma has been in an accident. Please pick up grandpa and take him to Valley Medical Center. I'll let him know. My boss is taking me now." My voice quivered as I spoke. I followed her out to the car, and she multi-tasked to drive and console me with my constant flow of tears.

At the hospital, I wasn't sure where to go. Emergency directed me to another counter and said a staff person would lead us where to go. My father and Ann arrived. Unable to see my mother, we were taken to a small room with chairs and a sofa. A woman came in and advised us emergency staff still had my mom. She would update us on the status of my mom's condition. I didn't like the scene of us in that room. It might as well have said, "Wait here until she dies."

My mom was on her walk in the neighborhood. Later I was informed she crossed a major intersection and was hit by a car, driven by a mother with her daughter. Within a few seconds, time stopped for my family.

I called my brother, Allen, who lived three hours away, to let him know. He worked long hard hours during that time, with a difficult work commute on highway 17 in the Santa Cruz Mountains.

"How bad is it? He asked.

"It doesn't look good. The hospital staff won't let us see Mom. She's still at emergency." I replied

Again, I asked to see my mom. We couldn't. My dad sobbed as his body shook all over. I held him and told him everything would be fine, but I knew better. Why did I tell him that? It wasn't going to be better. He knew too. The only time he ever cried was when he drank, he showed us affection by a hug, and told us he loved us.

She was his love, his sweetheart he cherished, and she felt the same way for him. I asked him once, "Daddy, why do you love Mom?"

"It's because of how she makes me feel," he replied.

He had a hard time expressing his feelings to us. While my mom left that afternoon, my dad made her favorite beef short rib and vegetable soup.

* * *

My mom was attractive, with a sense of style and poise. She met my dad, Mito, in the forties. She worked in a theatre and watched old movies with beautiful dancers. She dreamed of having children she could groom to teach the finer things in life. She was a Catholic who went to church every Sunday. She made sure we went to Catholic school. She taught us how to be faithful, loving, and giving people. She always said, "If somebody is mean to you. You don't have to be mean in return. Treat them with kindness."

Her fun-loving nature loved to entertain my friends, and they loved her. She never wanted to miss a party.

We had a very special relationship, and talked every morning. She listened and knew every part of my life in school and as an adult. Well, almost everything, some things are not meant for parents. She kept my brother and me busy. Although, there were times I saw a different side of her, the hot Latin temper when my dad wanted to be young and go out with his friends.

My aunt once told me many years ago, "I used to envy your mom; she had the most natural, sexy beauty about her." Of course, I saw her pictures. She projected a sense of confidence, beauty, and sass. She had a natural, Hispanic tan, long black licorice hair, hazel eyes, and a curvaceous body. She was born in Central California.

* * *

She called me that morning, and I didn't get the chance to return her call. It still haunts me. Even though my mother knew how much I loved her, it still hurt I didn't make that call. She usually called every morning. Sometimes to ask, "Are you ready for work? Did you have breakfast? I read the paper. There's an article on page two. It's in the business section. You should read it."

"Thanks, Mom, I'm running late. Talk to you later. Love you."

I needed someone to talk to, but I couldn't call Mark. I already let out my emotions at work and in the car on the way to the hospital. I had to keep it together for my family. If I called Mark, I would have lost it with more emotions.

I called my new friend, Mitch. He knew the staff at the hospital. He came right away, but he didn't say much. His serious face and stiff body language indicated my mom was in critical condition and fighting for her life. My ex-husband and his new girlfriend came to give Ann and our family support. It touched me they came. My two best friends, Jane and Joanne, and their spouses were also there.

"Mom, did you call Mark? You should." Ann said. She saw on my face I hadn't.

"No," I replied.

"You need to call him," she said.

"As soon as I know what's going on." I knew I should.

While we waited, the staff person came back. She told us they were taking our angel for a CAT scan and to watch the hallway. Soon, we saw her rolled by on the gurney. Her head tilted our way with her eyes open. I cried, "I love you."

She didn't respond, but I'm sure she heard.

We all sat in that little room, lit by overhead fluorescent lights, a table lamp, and a telephone and a Kleenex box lay on the table. It was enough room for seven of us to sit on the sofa and chairs. I can't remember many conversations except everyone wondering how it happened.

My boss came back to the hospital and left my car. She walked me to the parking lot to show me where my car was parked. I got inside the car to pull myself together before I went back in. Things unraveled in my head, I was confused and devastated. My father was very fragile. I cried while internal voices shouted for my attention with all the things needed.

Those voices shouted: He can't make it alone. How will you make it? Until finally, a peaceful voice said: Be still and strong.

At 5:30 p.m. on November 20, 1998, the social worker came in. I imagine everyone's head popped up as mine did, and we watched and listened to her slow, compassionate words, "Your wife and mother passed away. She had internal bleeding from the impact to her pelvis, which took her life. I'm going to give you a few minutes. Then another representative or I will discuss a few things with you."

God took our angel to heaven and found a perfect place for her. I got closer to my dad. He trembled with another flow of tears. I hugged him, and my daughter and I didn't let go. The hospital caregiver came in.

"Would you like a priest to give your mom a blessing? She asked.

"Yes, when will he come?" I asked.

"He's here. It won't be long," the caregiver replied.

I called Mark right after and told him everything. He cried on the phone and said he was sorry. He wanted to come right over. I told him we were waiting for the priest. I asked him to please give us an hour, then to meet us at my dad's house.

We walked into the hospital room while my mom lay on the bed. A sheet covered her petite body with only her face visible. The cold, clinical-looking room with a long counter on one side and overhead cabinets had dim lights, not as bright as some hospital rooms. My dad, daughter, and friends followed me in. Shortly after, the priest walked in. We all stood in a circle around my mom. I couldn't believe this motionless, stiff body was my mom, and at the same time, it wasn't her. It was like I watched a horrible scene in a movie. Not my mom, but a corpse.

"I'm sorry for your loss," the priest said. He began to say The Lord's prayer.

We later arrived at my parents' house that evening. My dad's out of town cousins came shortly thereafter to support him. I got drinks for everyone when I heard a knock at the door. I opened it, but couldn't see through the screen. Dark without the porch light on, Mark said, "It's me, Jean." I opened the door to let him in, and we hugged.

"Oh, Mark, I'm glad you're here." He walked in and greeted my dad, his cousins, and hugged my father. It meant everything to see him. He followed me into the kitchen.

"Mark, I'm taking my dad to my house for a while. So he won't be alone." I whispered.

"Jean, that's a great idea. I'll be there for you in any way. I love you." He hugged me again.

I knew financially; it would be difficult for my dad to manage things alone. My mom always handled business stuff. I needed time to think it over, so I helped him get clothes, and invited him to stay with me.

After my mom's sudden death, I thought I had gone through the toughest struggle in my life. I was a strong person. But, how would I hold myself together for my dad, in spite of my grief?

The woman who drove was not cited for killing my mom. Beyond angry, I kept going over it in my head. I tried to re-create the scene of how it happened. They said she wasn't on a crosswalk. I pictured my mom crossing the street to go to her favorite thrift store. She would buy a small trinket. The closest crosswalk was a block away. How could they not see her? Unless they turned onto the street and didn't pay attention to all sides. I requested the authorities to ask the women for a letter of forgiveness. It wasn't until I received the letter that I tried to forgive them.

A hole remained in my heart with my mom gone. I didn't know it at the time, but God's plan for phase one just happened. I figured out how to plan my mom's service, something I had never done. Were my signs coming to help me? But I couldn't see them yet.

I lived with my parents the year before she passed. I didn't renew the tenant's lease on my home and decided to move back in. In anticipation, I hired someone to paint both the inside and outside. I remember asking my mom, "How do you like the new colors?"

"I love what you did!" Mom said. I didn't know it at the time, but the house served as the hosting place after my mom's service a few months after I moved back in.

On the day of the services, I floated from one thing to the next, like an out of body experience. I wanted to be invisible. At the same time, I grieved the loss of my mom and tried to give support to my dad in making decisions. I wanted to scream, cry, and laugh, all at the same time. Emotions, unlike anything I experienced. My mask told everybody I was strong, but I felt detached from it all. My new friend, Mitch, attended and didn't know anyone but me. Mark was there and talked to all my family. I wanted to run and hide.

Even though we grieved my mom's passing to Heaven, an end to her physical being, it began a new relationship with dad. We became closer, more bonded in a way never before happened, and I wouldn't have imagined. He opened his heart, and believe it or not, I think he never opened up before, or I never heard him before.

During that time, I never lost communication with Mark. He called and checked in, and I appreciated his calls. In the evenings, I heard my father weeping in his new bedroom. I tried to comfort him. How could this be happening? Night after night, with good reason, he was in pain. We both were. I missed communicating with my mom. We talked about almost anything; she was my sounding board. Often she came to spend the night. She offered to help me around the house, with laundry or anything, but we just enjoyed the small slumber party of one night together. Often I heard her soft snore, a slight breath sound of, "Pu." The realization of her gone difficult to fathom.

This late cold winter evening, my dad and I tried to adjust to the chill of my mom's absence, without her cozy warmth and giggle. Then, of all times, my heater stopped working. Since I couldn't get a serviceman, in a panic, I called PGE to see if they could assist. They sent out a tall utility serviceman. He knocked at my front door, and I invited him to my home. His advice, "Ma'am, get a repairman. Keep the gas stove burners on all night."

My dad slept in the living room at the adjacent wall next to the kitchen. Even though the PGE man said it was safe, and it helped keep the home warm, I couldn't sleep. I tossed and turned and thought the house would burn down.

The next day when I called a repairman who inspected and said, "Ma'am, your heater crashed. There's a cover over the unit at the side. It's blocked at the vents and needs to be replaced."

"Oh, gosh! When can you replace it?" I said.

SECTION 1 - MARK & JEAN

"Ma'am, I need to check with my boss to see the schedules," he replied.

I wanted to cry. My dad stood there and listened, with his eyebrows raised.

"I have a few dollars I can loan you." My dad offered as he put his hand on my shoulder.

"That's okay, daddy, I'll try to work something out with the company. I'll tell them about mom, and maybe they'll let me make payments. Thank you, but don't worry."

Well, I worried but hoped we would be relieved in some way. I called the company owner and told them about my situation. They sounded empathetic and kind and allowed me to make three partial payments.

Overwhelmed with the weight of the decisions, both mentally and financially, I went to bed. I fell asleep and awakened at 3:00 a.m. In my dream: I saw myself at a party, carefully placing an assortment of berries on a silver tray, then carried the heavy tray in a room filled with people I didn't recognize. The chatter and laughter I heard quieted when someone accidentally bumped into me, and the tray fell to the floor. Suddenly, I heard my mom's voice, "That's okay, Jean, everything's going to be all right." I heard her in the room. My mom loved berries and made preserves and pies. It was real; I opened my eyes and started to cry.

I know God gave my mom a pass to talk to me, which was a blessing.

In the room, next door, my dad's hearing loss prevented him from hearing my wailing. I lay there in bed in the dark, surrounded by pillows behind my head, one on each side, and one between my knees. I wanted to talk to Mark. My internal conflict - One voice told me I needed to call him, with another saying I shouldn't. He was the first person I wanted to hear, so I leaned over to the nightstand, turned on the light, and called him. "Mark, I just had a dream and heard my mom's voice as if she was here," said with my broken words and tears.

"Oh, Jean! I wish I could hold you right now."

"I'm sorry I woke you."

"Do you want me to come over?"

"No, I'll be okay. It just seemed like she was here in my room, loud and clear. I miss her so much."

The way he comforted me convinced me I loved him. I tried to pull myself together, then I leaned out of bed and went to the bathroom. I didn't give up on him and our estranged relationship. I allowed myself time for him to settle his family issues, and hoped he would realize he couldn't live without me. We continued to communicate, but my life remained very busy with two jobs and the care of my father.

As time went on, as much as I loved my father, he began to treat me like a high school student, telling me what I should be doing from time to time. I knew I had to find him some social activities. I began to watch for senior activities in the newspaper. I called senior groups for suggestions. Young enough and healthy, I wanted him active again, so that he could move on.

I made arrangements in a men's support group, which met weekly for breakfast. A year since my mom passed, I helped him transition into a new social life.

One morning I read my local newspaper in the senior section highlighting weekly dance activities. I remembered what a great dancer he was at family events. He danced with me, doing the jitterbug, turning me, and I loved it. I showed him the article and suggested he try it out. Little did I know what I started!

By this time, I got him a private line with a voice mail and showed him how to retrieve his messages. One evening at dinner, not only could I see his Grecian formula, I smelled his strong after-shave cologne. I asked him, "Daddy, Are you going somewhere?"

"I'm going to have a few drinks, and maybe go to the dance," he said while he looked down.

"Oh, that's great! I think you'll enjoy it. Go shake your stuff!" I said. He laughed and hardly looked up.

As the weeks went by, he didn't go to the weekly breakfast. I did see that his phone recorder was blinking. One morning, he said to me, "Jean, can you check my messages, I forgot how to do it?"

Shocked and happy when I listened to the three women, who left messages for my dad. They said, "Mito, you are a great dancer… Please call me at…" Mito, I loved talking to you. Please call me … " Mito, I'd like to see you again, my number is … " After all, when dressed, the handsome, debonair man had a good sense of humor. I smiled as I delivered the messages of invitations to this hunk of a man, my dad, who the ladies wanted. He couldn't help but let out a hearty giggle himself. He still had a life to live. He was vibrant and transitioning to a new normal.

SECTION 1 - MARK & JEAN

SECTION 1 - MARK & JEAN

Chapter 5: Destiny
[1999 - 2000]

In 1999, I no longer felt safe and secure in the first home I purchased as an independent woman after my divorce in 1984. I loved this charming older home, but not the alley in the back and the detached garage. Also, my purse contents, including my driver's license, were stolen while at my office. My heavy purse sat underneath my desk and at the end of the day was empty.

Although I had sentimental reasons for not selling the house, I decided to sell it.

Reflecting on this, and the fact Mark wouldn't commit to a long term relationship, I made lifelong decisions. I told myself if I was going to grow old alone, it was okay, I would be fine, but I needed to live in a gated community.

Mark's friends watched and thought he was crazy to let me go. At the same time, they witnessed the painful, nasty divorce with his self-absorbed ex-wife. He confided to me how his ex-wife turned their friends against him with lies. He said she had fits of uncontrollable yelling, then turned and was charming. During his marriage, he never knew what he would get from day to day, tiptoeing in a field of flowers or minefields. He never left her, as he didn't want to leave his kids. He became complacent and numb to the relationship. He lost the passion to hunt and fish, which was his salvation. Then the bomb dropped when she left him. She told lies about Mark to justify why she left. He was shocked and disappointed. No wonder he was gun-shy.

Nevertheless, my attitude changed, and I thought I was okay without him and became his friend. I still thought of the fun times we had. Was it healthy to keep things going? He didn't want to get married?

At the time, I worked two jobs, during the week at a bank, and on the weekends on a real estate subdivision selling homes. I asked my weekend boss if I could work extra hours. I needed money for a larger deposit to buy one of the homes in his gated community.

SECTION 1 - MARK & JEAN

Mark came to see me at work on Sunday. He walked in with a thermos box, packed with my favorite things for lunch, a turkey and salami sandwich, salt and vinegar chips, iced tea, and chocolate chip cookies, his favorite. After lunch, I tested the waters again.

"Mark, I love my house, but I'm selling it. Since I was robbed, I don't feel safe. I need to sell. Whoever stole my purse knows where I live. I'm buying a home in a gated community. I'll feel safer."

"I don't blame you." He said with a look of concern.

After I heard his reply, it was hopeless. I thought he might have asked me to live with him for our future. I put my house on the market, and it sold quickly.

I continued to date Mark, but not exclusively, I gave up on him as a potential life partner. I probably seemed aloof and challenging. Mark began to pursue me differently and asked me to events out of town, but I declined. "We're not exclusive. I can't go out of town with you." I said.

* * *

In April 2000, depressed over my breakup with Mark, one of my girlfriends talked me into meeting her for brunch in Fresno.

"Quit acting sad. Act like you don't care. Make him miss you."

I took her advice. I continued dating others to get over Mark. A roller coaster of feelings, until I mentally pictured my new home and me moving into it alone. I gave up the idea of marriage; it seemed so far away from him.

After a few months, the chase was on again. He wanted me, and he didn't want to continue doing things alone with his friends. He invited me to dinner one evening at a Mexican restaurant, a close neighborhood watering hole, nothing fancy. We walked in early evening and sat at a booth in the bar, and one other couple sat with a sports station on the TV. The short middle-aged curly-haired bartender came over and asked us what we wanted.

"A margarita on the rocks, with salt," I said.

"Can you bring us a pitcher? How many drinks are in the small pitcher?" Mark asked.

"About five drinks," the bartender said.

SECTION 1 - MARK & JEAN

"Great! Bring it on!" Mark squeezed my hand.

This was unusual, he never ordered a pitcher. Like before, we had great conversations and laughter, but this was different. Salted rimmed glasses delivered with the pitcher, we toasted each other and had two drinks.

In the middle of my story, he interrupted and said what I hoped to hear for months.

"Jean, I want you to be my wife!"

"Do you know what you are saying?" I replied with laughter.

"Yes, I want you to be my wife!"

"Don't you think you should ask me?" I couldn't believe it!

"Will you marry me?"

"Yes!" I leaned toward him and kissed him. I honestly couldn't believe this happened.

"I say yes, but I think we better write this on a paper for proof." He laughed, as I tore a corner piece off of the scalloped green paper mat underneath our plates, while I put my other hand in my purse and reached for a pen.

"I don't have a ring, but we can go tomorrow and pick one out." So together, we wrote we would marry each other and dated it May 22, 2000.

In the meantime, he made a ring out of a tied, twisted napkin and put a large ice cube on top, the happiest moment I experienced in many years. Mark was my soulmate. My friend, Conn, knew it from the start. It took my absence from him to discover we were meant for each other.

Our friends lived near the restaurant, so we called them. They invited us to come for a celebratory drink, and we walked next door and toasted our happiness and engagement. Large fragrant magnolia blossoms were picked and set on their coffee table.

He kept his promise, and the next day we picked my engagement ring. He waited for two and a half years to finally decide to marry me. He didn't want to wait to plan a church wedding. I had six months to plan this wedding, but I didn't care, I waited for seventeen years to meet the right man. I never settled and waited for the right guy. Many emotions ran through me. I couldn't call my mom in Heaven, but silently I talked to her.

SECTION 1 - MARK & JEAN

I called my daughter Ann, my dad, Mito, and my aunt, Terry, my mom's sister, who was like my sister.

No doubts about our love but wondered if it would be strong enough for the family dynamics of a second marriage. I trusted and took the chance.

After waiting many years for the right person to marry my soul mate and favorite person, God finally got us together. Everything fit into place for the first time. I began to know it was such a beautiful perfect union and in every sense of the traditional mantra of the vows

"I take you for my lawful [wife/husband], to have and to hold, from this day forward, for better, for worse, for richer, for poorer, in sickness and health, to love and to cherish, until death; do us part."

I didn't know how much more deeply I would love and cherish him in those last few years.

Even though everyone knows you marry for love, you need to be especially cautious in the legal nature of a second marriage in protecting your livelihood and financial matters relating to adult children in both marriages. My fiancé had more separate assets because he shared that information with me. I wasn't interested in his portfolio. I had my retirement, but at the same time had to protect my future in the house, as I would be contributing money to the household. I had a financial background and saw many portfolios and knew to protect myself.

Before we married, Mark asked if I wanted to buy a new home or if I wanted to move into his home, it was larger than my new home. I decided to move into his home because it was modest, well-located, and affordable. Since I was contributing half of the expenses to our new household, I requested that if he died before me, the home come to me free of any debt. I did not want to buy another home. He agreed and purchased a term life insurance policy to pay off the mortgage should he die first. I had no other requests and felt satisfied and secure he agreed.

God had His plan. Our intimate wedding ceremony was at the small chapel of a Baptist church in Fresno, California, in October 2000. We were husband and wife, after the ups and downs of our courtship for two and a half years. Mark finally got over his tumultuous divorce and trusted me. Even though financially in different places of our life, he could retire, slow down and travel more, I was in a different place, I still worked. That was okay, it was about us, not the things.

Since this was our second marriage, we went against the traditional ways. I was escorted down the aisle in a simple ivory dress by my two grandsons, James and Thomas, ages four and six. Young and handsome, the boys were also bright enough and good-natured enough to be trusted to give their grandmother away. James, the older, looked more like my side of the family, with thick dark brown hair and dark brown eyes and was a bit shy. Thomas, the younger, had lighter brown hair, blue eyes, and a fearless personality. In his gray suit, Mark was escorted by his two adult daughters, both tall and beautiful. They lived out of town, and I had not spent much time with them but was hopeful for the future.

Mark's brother, Robert, was his best man, and my daughter, Ann, was my matron of honor. She wore an iridescent violet-colored dress. My dad had a place of honor in front to give me away.

While we looked at each other and smiled, I tried to keep tears from falling, as the preacher said to me, "Do you promise to love him, comfort him, honor and keep him for better or worse, for richer or poorer, in sickness and health and forsaking all others, be faithful only to him so long as you both shall live?" We both said our 'I do's.'

"Please congratulate Mr. and Mrs.!" Mark kissed me and then threw his hands in the air and yelled out, "Woo Hoo!"

All the family and friends knew I waited for almost seventeen years for my prince, and Mark knew he could be himself with me, and everyone saw how happy he was. He gave me love and attention. He listened to me and made me laugh.

We hosted a small lunch reception of 50 guests at our neighborhood golf country club on the river bluff in Fresno. We were serenaded by our musician, Maurisco, who played soft guitar songs, as he moved among the tables. A perfect setting with the sun gently filtered through the windows, which highlighted the table centerpieces of white and purple orchid plants. The grandchildren and younger cousins made friends, laughed, and moved around the tables. The adults moved from table to table socializing after eating lunch of vegetarian lasagna and salads. Mark and I sat at the center with smiles celebrating our time, while everyone watched the toasting of champagne and the cutting of the strawberry-filled white wedding cake.

Late October, fall changed colors of red, to amber and toast. The air was crisp and fresh, and nothing could have been better. Mark planned a beautiful drive from Vancouver to Victoria Island. We saw the cultural island history, tasted the historic tea and biscuits at the Empress Hotel, dined at the finest restaurants, and walked the promenade along the Harbour, on Victoria, B.C. to Port Angeles, WA.

* * *

I didn't know it, but a few years later, after we were married, Mark began to lose his way, often repeating himself, then misplacing things and drifting from time and place with his memory. My heart was in my throat. He unintentionally canceled the policy.

I loved him so much. I loved him more than I could stand it.

SECTION 2 - DOCTORS & MEMORY LOSS

Chapter 6: Signs & First Visit
[2005]

The signs Mark suffered from memory loss surfaced in 2005, about five years after our marriage.

In preparation for one of his fishing or adventure trips, Mark often silently intense, looked after every detail. Methodically, he started two to three weeks ahead, slowly brought stuff into his man cave, which doubled as his home office. Each adventure unique; hunting, fly fishing, freshwater, or deep-sea fishing, took him to Wyoming, Montana, Oregon, Alaska, British Columbia, Mexico, and Costa Rica. A vast collection of every furry lure and heavyweight, the proper rods and reels for fishing, and rifles for hunting were on hand. He kept almost everything locked in the garage in a large safe, a metal cabinet, and an extra storage unit. The weather conditions dictated how he outfitted himself. He had light or heavyweight camouflage vests, hats, jackets, boots, and waders.

Mark selected the lines needed ahead of time. Great care was taken to make sure no tangles were in the line and would stream through the reel with ease. The rainbow selection of pink (faded red), blue, green, and yellow colors of line dictated which color meant for the depths of water they would fish. Rods and reels, every one of them on the floor, inspected and cleaned, giving each one equal time and consideration. The travel and tackle bags held water repellent hats, and shirts were sun screened. It was a ceremony. Which item or piece of gear was lucky enough to spend the entire trip with him? I always chuckled when I watched him. His forehead furrowed in concentration, and he rubbed his hands or his scalp as if he stored ideas. He whistled throughout the house when satisfied.

On his trips, Mark often dressed in his favorite hunting gear. It consisted of a signature red and black checkered flannel shirt, jeans, a tan suede vest, leather hunting boots, and a canvas safari hat, like a harmonious Cardinal, hard to dismiss with striking, fiery, red feathers on the songbird.

SECTION 2 - DOCTORS & MEMORY LOSS

In September 2005 he seemed different and more confused in the home office almost all day, and he took longer to prepare. He forgot what he packed and then emptied a bag or case to repack. He drove to the storage unit more than once. Back at home, he unpacked again and found it already packed. I didn't give it a second thought. He had so much out, and I couldn't imagine myself remembering it all. I wanted to distract him and take him away. I thought, Maybe we can go out to dinner.

"I hope you get this excited on our next trip!" I said.

"Of course!" he replied.

He knew his equipment, he fished and hunted since his grandfather was alive. He made these trips since he was in college about forty years ago. He also had friends for every one of those occasions. This particular trip to San Francisco with a friend's husband, Jude. So off, Mark and Jude went deep sea fishing.

After the trip, Mark returned home and said, "One of my boxes of lures is missing. Either someone took it, or I left it on the boat."

My girlfriend told me later - her husband Jude told her - Mark looked for his fishing tackle and lost his balance. Distracted, he almost fell off the boat and needed help to hold him back. This scared me. He could have fallen in the ocean.

I grew quite concerned. It didn't sound like Mark. I knew he needed to retire, and I was glad he had semi-retired. We had one more large real estate job to complete at work. I didn't know if stress over the job or if something else was happening. Maybe he could retire after it was finished.

The following Monday, Mark and I stood in our offices and discussed when it would be safe to leave the office, due to mockingbirds attacking us as we walked outside. We became nervous to leave the office. We couldn't see where they hid, but as soon as we opened the door, they charged at us. Think of the movie The Birds by Alfred Hitchcock, and it felt that way!

The office phone rang. I answered Mark's previous office partner and handed the phone to Mark. As I listened, stress lines deepened on Mark's face. His voice was high, confused, and agitated. He had transitioned to part-time work, but after I heard this conversation, I had to talk him into full retirement. He hung up the phone and said, "I'm pissed. He said I

SECTION 2 - DOCTORS & MEMORY LOSS

didn't state everything he needed on the real estate report, and I left things out of the report."

I didn't know what to say, so I kept silent. Did Mark make a mistake with the report? Is he embarrassed or even aware of the mistake?

I looked at the display on the office walls, wood, and gold plaques, given to him by community organizations. Previously, over eight days, together, we moved all his thirty-plus years of real estate files from the old office to this new one. We thought it time to down-size, and also, we wanted to have our own office together. How could he be changing so quickly?

Will I be able to continue working without him if he has to retire completely? What is happening? To him? To us?

I put my hand on his shoulder as he sat at his desk. The worry on his face killed me.

"Why don't I talk to your assistant, who typed the report, and we'll try and figure it out?" I said soothingly.

"Okay," he said while he looked bitter.

I decided to change the topic. Get both of our minds off things. "More importantly, how the hell are we going to get out of here without getting our faces clawed off?"

The diversion worked. Mark seemed to think about me first, our safety. He reverted as a protector.

"I'll go first," he said, "then you follow. Put a file folder in front of your face. Call the property manager to see if they will come to help us." I did. Then I followed his lead. I thought, how can they help us?

We pulled together, protective shields over our faces, and quickly ran out the door. Never had we experienced mockingbirds charging at us before. It was scary, their beaks smashed and tapped onto the folder in front of our faces, and their wings brushed and flapped our heads. We made it to the car and dove inside like terrified rabbits. But I was more worried about Mark. He was confused and stressed.

While we waited in the car for the property manager, I thought about the red flags of Mark's actions recently, and I noticed strange conversations. Sometimes he'd recall a statement I made, but mixed up. He said I said something else. I repeated answers to a question, over and over. When I mentioned my concern, he rationalized, "Lots of people my age are forgetful."

This was true, but I knew different. He's in trouble. Something is wrong. He's in denial.

His family knew it too. They witnessed the signs of his memory problems, but I respected his wishes not to tell anyone. Over the months and years, he was adamant I kept it secret. This added to the strain with his daughters, and the influence of their mother, his ex-wife. I knew they thought I married their dad for money. I kept his secret, even though I tried to tell him everyone loved him and needed to know, including his close friends. I told him it could happen to anyone, and I'd be with him to the end no matter what. In the back of my mind, I fantasized about a miracle drug to help him. Truthfully, I felt cheated.

The property manager phoned and was delayed, so we went home. I focused and kept my mind on driving. It was late when we got home, so we went to a drive-through for dinner. I felt guilty when I didn't cook, but later we ate turkey-burgers. I searched Google for Dementia and Alzheimer's. Everything I read said to exercise, socialize, eat right and get proper sleep, all to prevent or slow down the illness. He did all those things. Why did this happen to him, to us? I began to feel like I had Dementia as well, exhausted and wiped out from fear I could barely press my fingers on the keyboard. Thinking about it at all left me both horrified and dead inside. Mark was leaving me. I could not save him.

* * *

My mind ran through past conversations and facts about his health from when we first met in 1997. He told me he wasn't as passionate about fishing and hunting. And he didn't have the same sexual drive. He thought it was from taking Melatonin, which helped him sleep after his divorce. He did the treadmill every day and lifted weights in his home office. We walked in the evenings for exercise. During those early times, I couldn't keep up with him. I remembered our skydive together that year. Magical. Would I ever get to feel alive with him again?

SECTION 2 - DOCTORS & MEMORY LOSS

* * *

He was sixty-four when I wanted Mark to go to the doctor, but he wouldn't go. Later that week, I was in the car at a real estate client's office. About ready to go in, his daughter Tammy phoned me. She said her dad called her repeatedly and forgot he already called her on the same day. My response to her, "I'll be a pushy broad and call the doctor." Mark also said to me on more than one occasion, "I called the girls. I don't know why they don't return my calls."

I never got out of the car at my client's office. I sat there and stared at the windshield. It felt like I had on heavy shoulder pads. I couldn't move or think. Part of me didn't want to think about it, and we had been married for five years. Yes, I felt selfish, but I wanted to ignore it. My heart pounded so fast, and it tapped the walls of my chest. The only person I could talk to and trust was my daughter Ann, but I didn't want to burden her either. I felt utterly and completely alone.

"Ann, it's Mom. Mark is forgetting things." I decided to come clean with her. I couldn't take it anymore on my own. Ann was home in Clovis, trying to get ready for work.

"What do you mean? Like forgetting to be somewhere on time?"

"No. It's more than that. I'm worried."

"Worried enough to see a doctor?"

"Yes, it's serious. His primary doctor referred us to a neurologist."

"Oh no."

"He doesn't remember times or places. He forgets the people we chatted with yesterday. There are gaps in his memory. He knows me but repeats questions. He's aware sometimes, and then he forgets things."

"That's awful. How are you?"

"Scared. Shitless."

* * *

In the car at the neurologist's office, waiting in the parking lot, Mark narrowed his eyes at me in the passenger seat. He slapped his thigh. "I

SECTION 2 - DOCTORS & MEMORY LOSS

don't want to go in. There's nothing wrong. Everybody my age forgets." He paused then said, "I am still working!"

"I know. Let's just see what this doctor says." I let him cool down and put my hand on his shoulder, and said, "What can it hurt?" He doesn't realize he's been making mistakes.

He glared at me as if I tortured him; and I didn't blame him. He didn't budge. But he should. Our appointment was too important. How will I ever get him inside?

Perspiration made itself present on my upper lip and neck, and I could see beads of sweat on his temples and forehead. I turned on the engine and the air conditioning before I reached in the back and pulled out a Kleenex to gently wipe his forehead and temples and dried myself.

"Let's give this a try. If you don't like it, we won't come back. Okay?"

"I guess."

I'm turning the engine off. It's gonna get hot again if we don't walk in." I opened my door and put one leg out. It was hot outside in Fresno. I'd worn a nice top and pants, and already every inch of fabric was soaked.

I finally got him inside the office and walked up to the granite reception counter. We were not acknowledged. None of the three receptionists even bothered to look up. From the looks of the other stoic couples in the cramped waiting room, it was obvious no one wanted to be recognized. The receptionist finally looked up. She handed us questionnaires and asked us to complete each one individually. She told us their team would interview us separately before we saw the doctor. As I held Mark's hand, we took a seat, and I asked, "Do you want some help filling out the form?" He nodded then looked at the others in the room. Mark seemed dazed, uncertain why we'd come to a doctor's office for memory problems. I expected him to get up and walk out. Luckily, he didn't do anything but sit and helped me answer questions.

With the clipboard on my lap, I scanned the forms and hurried. The questions started with:

Why did I contact the doctor?
What behavior changes have I noticed?
How is his overall health?
How does this make me feel?

Is he on a diet?

Is he taking any supplements?

Does he work out regularly?

On and on. The questions kept coming. I leaned over and whispered in Mark's ear, "I'll be right back. I'm going to the reception counter."

I whispered to the receptionist. "Am I allowed to help my husband with his questionnaire?"

"Only help out with the social security numbers, your address, and phone number. Let him complete what he can on his own. The interviewer will help. He meets separately in a few minutes," she said. She turned to assist another patient.

I walked back. Leaned over to Mark and whispered, not to worry about the questions he couldn't answer. He would get help during the interview. He rolled his eyes, then shook his head. In a few minutes, a young man with a pleasant-looking face called Mark. Mark looked at me and asked if I was going with him. I shook my head, indicating he needed to go alone. I felt he might question it, but he got up and followed the man.

My entire body shook. I had to pull myself together and stop being worried about a diagnosis I wasn't sure was true.

In a few minutes, a plump nurse in a blue uniform walked out and called my name. I followed her into a wide hallway, funneled into a small office with a desk. I sat with this stranger, apprehensive as hell. Growing up, my parents always told me to keep personal things at home. My eyes teared, and my mouth watered. I worried about Mark in his private interview.

The nurse put bottled water on the desk. With a slight smile, she said, "This is for you." She held the questionnaire. Her thick-lensed glasses with wide black frames appeared heavy and laid low on her nose. She held the page firmly with her left hand while her right index finger moved down the page. Then she flipped to the next pages and repeated. Somehow, as I watched her, it gave me a sense of comfort. She knew what she was doing, and she didn't seem nervous, upset, or worried. Her calm demeanor, of a wife and mother of kids, made me somehow feel better and stronger. I made it up. I truly knew nothing about her. Yet, her energy seemed caring and kind.

SECTION 2 - DOCTORS & MEMORY LOSS

She nodded. "I can tell from your answers; you've been through some changes. How do you feel about all these changes?" She settled the papers while she looked at me with compassionate brown eyes.

I decided to be truthful and to let all of my bottled-up emotions spill out a little at a time. "It's upsetting. I want to cry and yell. We got married in 2000. We've been married for almost six years. Mark's in denial about his memory loss and doesn't want me to tell anyone, not even his children. His daughters have noticed it, and the youngest daughter told me he repeats calls to her, saying the same thing over again within a few minutes. His primary doctor thinks it is mild cognitive impairment."

The kind nurse nodded. "The doctor will evaluate his cognition by asking him to perform simple things to see where he is. Don't worry. I'll walk you back to the waiting room, so you can be there when Mark comes back. Then, I'll return and get both of you for the meeting with the doctor."

"Okay." I wiped my eyes with the backs of my hand. "Thanks for your help." I followed her through the hallway and took a seat. Within a few minutes, Mark came out and sat next to me. I smiled at him, held his hand, and kissed him on the cheek.

"We'll talk later," I whispered.

As we waited, I watched Mark try to read a magazine. He glanced back and forth at others and looked back down quickly. He seemed uneasy like he didn't want anyone to notice him, which felt impossible in that setting. Most of the others in this waiting room appeared much older than us. Mark was sixty-four years old. I was fifty-six.

Many minutes passed after the separate interviews when the same plump nurse in her blue uniform walked out and called us. As I picked up my purse, Mark looked at me, and I held his hand as we walked together. We followed her into the hallway, and she told us to take the door on the right. The doctor greeted Mark with a handshake, then turned to me. At my petite size, the doctor and I were at eye to eye level. With a commanding voice, he told us to please take a seat. The doctor remained standing with a stiff body, chin up and arms folded, as we both sat lower than him.

He didn't mince words. "Based on the test results, Mark has Early Cognitive Impairment. It will probably turn into Alzheimer's." Mark and I looked at each other stunned. My mouth watered, and I swallowed. Mark, who was normally tan, looked drained of color. His face went chalk-white.

"Are you sure?" I asked.

"Don't a lot of people my age start getting forgetful?" He said rudely. I knew he was terrified.

"This is different from the forgetful you're thinking of." The doctor pushed our file across his desk. "It's not only short-term memory but also cognitive thinking. Ways of thinking are different and confused. Some people get this as early as their forties. We can start some medication to slow it down, but there's no cure. I'll write you a prescription for Aricept and give you some sample pills to help get you started." The doctor started writing. I watched Mark, and I could see the muscles in his cheek contracting. At the same time, I felt my face tightening. I didn't know who would erupt first, but I tried to take a deep breath. The doctor delivered his message in an impersonal manner, like a tin robot. I imagined he said the same message daily to other patients. I realized he couldn't get drawn into the emotions, but where was his heart? The least he could have shown us was an empathetic smile.

He handed me the prescription and I don't remember saying thank you. We left the waiting room, out the door into fresh hot air. Both hanging onto each other as if the ground rolled beneath us.

Mark said, "I didn't like him. I'm not going back there!"

"Let's not worry about that now. We can get another referral for a new neurologist from our primary doctor. We'll get one more opinion."

"This is crap."

"I know, honey. I know."

After I heard the doctor's awful, devastating news, I drove us to St. Anthony's Catholic church. We walked into the lobby. I tapped my fingers in the holy water, placed them on my forehead, and moved them with the sign of a cross. Mark followed my actions. As we went into the main sanctuary, I smelled a scent of incense with a piney, sweet, woody aroma. I placed my purse on the wooden pew and took some money out. I folded my dollars flat, so they fit in the tin money box on the wall. Sticks stood in a small sandbox in front of all the glass jars holding the candles.

Some were lit, some unlit. I reached for one stick, then touched a lit candle and lit another one.

Mark watched me as I walked over to him. I sat, and he gently squeezed my thigh. I know he was scared; we both were. I didn't know what the future looked like with this diagnosis. I felt alone, miserable and I wanted to bawl. I wanted to throw something and scream at God. Instead, I sat there, trying to be braver than I ever was in my life. Mark didn't want me to share this with his family.

I looked over at the candles and reflected how a lit candle was my lifeline. It was always the way I took extra time to ask God for help or to thank him. While the sun filtered in from the stained-glass windows, we sat, and I watched the colorful lines reflecting on the walls of the church. I took a deep breath, pursed my lips, and thought, I know you are here, God, can I lean on you?

I knelt with my arms rested on the back of the pew in front of me and stared at the large crucifix and began to think of everything I had done wrong. Why was this happening to us? We were newly married, on our way to an amazing life together. It had to be a mistake. The diagnosis was wrong. The doctor was an ass. In my way, without talking, I asked God for forgiveness. It was how I'd learned from early childhood to get his attention. Ask Him for forgiveness. I crossed my arms and lay my head down.

* * *

Our life turned upside down with Mark's Early Onset Dementia, which becomes Alzheimer's it was incurable and morphed him into a zombie. Easygoing Mark teeter-tottered into his new normal; being combative and yelling profanities. He flipped from being with me like he'd always been to off in his own dark, private world. With a vacant yet preoccupied look on his face, Mark saw invisible people and was invaded by internal terrorists. He looked blank and dull with no expression as he stared into the open space of another world only he could see, a world not visible to me. It frightened me, but I went along.

"Mark?" I asked him once. "What do you see?"

"What are you talking about?" he answered blank-eyed.

"What do you see when you stare off into space?"

He didn't answer. He had no idea what I asked. I thought, never mind, I was afraid to know.

Still, Mark was Mark. He would always be my Mark. His eyes revealed love, true gut-wrenching love, the real love and faith between us giving me purpose. I would never leave him. No matter what happened.

That being said, I wasn't perfect. There were many days where the only thing that helped me was when I said, "Fuck! Oh, God, why?" For which I had to perform a thousand Hail Mary's.

Simultaneously, I continued to daydream of the life we had before he got sick. The warm memory of travels, hiking, and entertaining with family and friends. Would six years together be enough to fill me? I moved in and out of our new normal, with a fast-shifting sunbeam of determination, and tried to keep remnants of our light. I often failed. I'd wake up in the morning, only to feel our precious time together was running out.

SECTION 2 - DOCTORS & MEMORY LOSS

SECTION 2 - DOCTORS & MEMORY LOSS

Chapter 7: Second Opinion
[2006]

Later in 2006, we got a second opinion. The new neurologist, a young to a middle-aged female doctor with short blond hair, allowed me in the room during Mark's analysis and testing. This doctor was very compassionate and thorough, and she asked Mark thirty verbal questions for recall and cognition. He was given a clipboard with paper and then asked to draw different shapes and objects, like a clock. Mark's responses may not have been correct, but he answered with ease. I watched him smile and could tell he liked her. He teased her and asked her if she could remember the same questions. Being present gave me an understanding of his mental ability and alertness during that doctor setting. In a way, he was his old self. I grappled with what it meant to see him changing. I longed him before, super smart, reliable, loving, and kind. Wasn't he forever and always the same person, illness, or no illness? Memory loss or not? I was envious as they laughed together at his easy banter. Would I have to intervene? Would I have to throw my precious husband under the bus and let the doctor know he wasn't always this way; easygoing, funny, the life of the party? My stomach clenched, and my hands filmed with sweat and a few unbroken tears formed in my eyes. I wanted to scream, 'and what about me? Who's going to help me?

Instead, I put on my sock puppet face, "Oh, he is quite the flirt when he wants to be," I chimed in with a great deal of aplomb as if it mattered. What was wrong with me? Was I so desperate to be recognized, acknowledged, included in their witty verbal repertoire'?

The doctor explained how the test was rated. Thirty was the highest and best score, and the lower scores meant a drop in his memory and cognitive abilities. After the test, the neurologist concurred he had mild cognitive impairment, called Early Onset Dementia. She offered another medication, Namenda, which might help. She encouraged Mark to go for further testing with doctors at the University of California, San Francisco Alzheimer's Center. Again, no cure for his illness, but she implied the medication might help improve by slowing down the process. Is this like terminal cancer? Just thinking of comparison-terminal made me want to throw up. I tried breathing slowly. I tried holding my breath. If someone held me forcibly underwater, it would have felt the same. Complete hopelessness and loss. Complete suffocation. I wanted to scream, "I need oxygen! ME-ME-ME!"

The doctor suggested I contact the Valley Caregivers Association for education about the illness. I needed to know what to do, how to treat him within the scattered confines of our new normal. So, I did. I was obedient to the letter. I stopped sleeping well. I believed I might never sleep well again, and often jerked awake to see that Mark was beside me. But which, Mark? The man I married, or another man, someone I no longer knew.

"Here I go," I mouthed continually, as if being obedient and prayerful, reciting the rosary ten times a day, would gain me points with God.

Hail Mary full of grace, the Lord is with thee.

Blessed are thou among women, and blessed is the fruit of thy womb Jesus.

Holy Mary Mother of God, pray for us sinners now and at the hour of our death. Amen.

…that we may be worthy of the promises of Christ.

A week later, I sat in Fresno in class with a cross-section of caregivers, mostly spouses, men, and women, who were 10 to 15 years older, few my age of fifty-seven years old. I dealt with an illness that typically attacked older victims, people well into their seventies, eighties, and nineties. Our new family, with the illness of our spouses or loved ones as a common denominator, kept anonymous and confidential names within our group. Honestly, I was so out of place. I wanted to shout, 'This isn't supposed to happen to me! To us! We've only been married for six years! We're too young! I DON'T BELONG HERE! I'm not one of YOU!' It felt like quicksand took me over, invading my eyes, nose, and mouth as I looked around the tiny room. There were fifteen participants, sniffling, sneezing, scooting inside their hard metal folding chairs. Yes, we all wore puffy, dark bags under our sad, glazed-over eyes, and our lips pursed with anger, regret, and terror. And while we had sick spouses, parents, or siblings in common, I couldn't grasp any of it. Why? That internal terrorist of horror, shame, and rage inside me would not go away. This dreaded disease, a

SECTION 2 - DOCTORS & MEMORY LOSS

death sentence, slowly ate away at my loved one's brain and body. The class started. People began talking. I learned about things I didn't want to remember, yet I had to understand what was happening to my husband. The list of causes of Dementia was endless. Other forms of Dementia stemmed from Parkinson's, Lewy Body, brain injuries, brain tumors, and Downs Syndrome.

Our moderator, a medium-sized Hispanic woman, wore a compassionate demeanor and smile. My mind told me to smile back, but sometimes I rebelled, sick of trying to act like a good little girl or wife. I wanted to pick up our chairs and throw them against the wall. I wanted to blame. BLAME-BLAME-BLAME-God, but no, I couldn't. It was our failed medical system to find a cure to this mind-rape of an illness, the environment, stupid people who tried to be caring or supportive, offering tips on Vitamin E capsules, like taking a hundred of them would result in a complete return to wellness rather than severe stomach cramps.

Little packets of chocolate chip cookies, crackers or peanuts, and small bottled waters neatly arranged at a front table along with pamphlets, as if it was a happy get-together or a little lunch party. We all listened, with an unspoken trust, to keep each and everyone's life private and personal. We spoke freely and openly about our loved ones and the trials we faced daily.

"My wife slapped me in the face yesterday," someone said. It was silent. I heard, but I wasn't ready to share just yet.

"My son ran out the front door. The cops looked for him for hours. He couldn't remember where he lived." Another one offered.

"If you don't already have alarms. I suggest to get them. And, add door monitors." The moderator added.

"Is anyone having trouble monitoring medications? A woman asked.

"We will have a speaker in two weeks. It's on medication management," said the moderator.

"I have to watch my husband, so he takes the pills," a woman yelled out.

In the same boat, as all participants in the room, treading in a lost unfamiliar place, I tried to adjust to the new culture of behavior I couldn't gauge or temper. Some of the illnesses mentioned, more than I imagined, mimicked each other. Consequently, none of us could ascertain

SECTION 2 - DOCTORS & MEMORY LOSS

the timing. It was difficult to organize the types of different behaviors, let alone categorize them as to when and how they befell our loved ones, and how and when they would unfold. The education provided by the local Valley Caregiving Organization helped, but didn't prepare me for everything ripped from under the foundation of our worlds.

Time and again, I thought I could stand it, and then I toppled down the unbearable rabbit hole, quicksand in my eyes, nose, and mouth.

A visit to his new neurologist revealed she had to report his illness to authorities.

"I have to report your condition to the DMV," his new neurologist said sweetly.

"What?" Mark asked. "What did you say?"

"The DMV. You might not be allowed to drive. They have to test you."

His face turned ashen. If he hadn't been seated in the exam room, I believe he would have needed to sink into a chair somewhere fast. The doctor reassured Mark he could still drive but he needed another test before his license could be reissued. He turned to me with watery eyes and said nothing. I know he feared he wouldn't pass the test, and worse yet, never drive again. This was an attack on his manhood, beyond what either of us could handle. He was my great adventurer, man. There was no way I could let him fail his driving test. What could I do? Who could I bribe? My mind wouldn't shut off with solutions so outlandish. I had to restrain myself from voicing them out loud. 'We have a house, I wanted to say to the neurologist. You can have it if you will forget we were here. Throw his file away. Burn it with gasoline and matches. Please don't tell the DMV.'

Shortly thereafter, Mark received a letter from the DMV asking him to return his current license unless he physically went to the local testing office to be retested. The day we sat at the DMV waiting for his driving test, it was burning hot in the small room. To match that intense heat, his face was red with stress and humiliation, only one other man sitting in the room. I wasn't sure if I wanted Mark to pass or not. My heart raced with worry. If he passed and hurt someone, what then? If he didn't pass and he dove into a deep depression, what then? Fortunate, or unfortunate, he passed the test and given his license. Not only did he pass, when he

SECTION 2 - DOCTORS & MEMORY LOSS

received his new license in the mail, the DMV, in error, renewed it for five years. It should have been renewed for only one year. A small victory perhaps. Yet didn't we deserve something good to happen? Wasn't this a 'Win?'

"Mark," I said, trying to helpful. "This is great. You can still drive."

"Can I?" he said. "How do you know?" We'd just been to the DMV. My heart looped like a whip inside my chest.

The new neurologist suggested I start offering to drive. It was an effort to get Mark used to the passenger seat. I did it. But, I was always fearful. He hated it. I hated it worse. Even though I drove miles for our real estate business, my teeth often clenched when I drove him around.

"Do you need more air?" I asked, trying to be helpful. "Do you want me to crack the window?"

"Why don't you just drive," he said, sullenly.

The years leading up to this invasion didn't prepare us for what we faced. The continued visits to teams of doctors, the inward denial of this ugly disease continued to invade him inwardly and outwardly, and the deception we both enacted like the biggest liars or bit-show actors in the world. At the same time, we tried to keep it secret from everyone. It was his solemn request of me, even though his family was really upset. I imagined witnessing his behavior. It was clear to them something wrong was happening to Mark.

It was a real test for both of us. As I look back at the years of Mark's physical deterioration, there was no way any book or person could have prepared us for what was in store. It was a gradual take-over of his old self and his pure spirit. The wonderful, fun-loving, adventuresome, peaceful man I married changed daily into a man possessed by this internal terrorist. I couldn't understand how it randomly destroyed his brain.

Strangely though, sometimes it felt like he was back to his old self, not his new self. He was highly alert, remembered dates and places not confused about any of his facts as he rattled them off. This atrophy, also called plaque, moved around his brain as though it hadn't permeated his brain. Amyloid plaques are one of the two brain abnormalities defining Alzheimer's disease (AD). The appearance of amyloid plaques in the brain

SECTION 2 - DOCTORS & MEMORY LOSS

can proceed to the behavioral symptoms by years. Amyloid plaques are sticky buildup that accumulates outside nerve cells or neurons.

At times his memory loss and the diagnosis of Alzheimer's felt like a phantasm, an illusion meant to trick us somehow; that it wasn't true. He had allergies; was this an allergic reaction to some substance in his brain? Why was he back sometimes and then not? I'll admit, that it was some form of denial, I mentally called off this invasive disease of my Mark's body and spirit, as if I had the power to wave a magic wand. I often prayed to myself, Please, dear God, help him and take it away.

In the beginning stages, I felt cheated and selfish. We'd both talked of spending more time together after our retirement with each other, our family, traveling, and creating. He suppressed his creative side to provide for his family in his first marriage. He hoped to paint. I hoped to write or draw.

As frustrated as I was from the fatigue of the ongoing care he needed, I began to love him more deeply each day. I felt God's hand guiding me; I couldn't do enough for him. It was as if he received the same message form his side of things, and he craved and wanted more of me. I was his caregiver.

Everything he did was at a child's pace, showered, and walked at a very slow pace. I witnessed such a daily confusing roller coaster of behavior. It was a familiar feeling to me, from my childhood and young adult years. Here I go up into the heavens, clink-clink-clink, and then whoosh, here I am falling to the ground.

Before I married Mark, I was a caregiver and a mediator for my parents, who struggled and needed me as a buffer. They went from loving and defending to bickering and criticizing each other. My mom was more of a homebody, and my father needed more. My mom's smile, giggly personality, and generosity drew people in, and everybody loved her, including my friends. My dad loved her with all his heart but had no patience for her secret spending. It would cause an avalanche of arguments each time.

Yes, my mom did have a compulsive spending problem. It nearly wiped out their funds. It harmed my dad, and it shook me. Roller coaster up, roller coaster down.

SECTION 2 - DOCTORS & MEMORY LOSS

In some way, it prepared me for the uncertainties of Mark's illness, not knowing what to expect from day-to-day. Mark was aloof and unpredictable. In the morning, when we lay in bed, I suggested a trip to the landscape nursery. He loved our discussions about gardening and the selection of flowers and plants during breakfast, though it changed when he drifted into another world. As soon as we got home and went outside, he lost the desire for gardening or planting.

I tried to entice him with a lawn chair outside the garage door. He sat and watched me for a few minutes with a preoccupied look, while I pruned roses in the front and cleaned out the flowerbed. It didn't last, and he walked back inside. I forged magic from nothing, and then slowly, Mark slipped away from me, leaving me outside to look at a bunch of roses with thorny stems I wanted to slice all over my arms.

Previously he loved going outside into the garage to clean things out. It was his excuse to talk to the neighbor friends and socialize. My adventure man was gone. If he was off having adventures, they were internal and bound by the laws of other universes, and none of them included me anymore.

And soon, another loved one was getting sick.

SECTION 2 - DOCTORS & MEMORY LOSS

SECTION 2 - DOCTORS & MEMORY LOSS

Chapter 8: Hospice Trial Run
[2008]

A slight chill in the air in February 2008, Mark and I walked inside from the garden. The phone rang from his brother, Robert. His mom fell and taken to the hospital. She already had Dementia, degenerative disk problems, and with this fall, more complications.

We arrived at the hospital. Mark's mom looked at us and smiled. Only after the relief from the pain meds could she smile, but the medication provided comfort, like a Band-Aid. At age 92, the doctor said they couldn't do surgery. It was time to find her a skilled nursing facility, and the discharge nurse suggested a list of names for the family to find a place.

"I'm so sorry, Mark," I said.

He was distant, cold, off somewhere in his other place of existence.

We visited his mom at the hospital the next morning. Mark's face was blotchy, deeply lined and pale beneath his eyes and nostrils. The short conversation demonstrated his confusion over his mom's condition. He repeated questions every twenty minutes or so.

"Is the medication helping her?"

"Is the medication helping her?"

"Is the medication helping her?"

Obvious to Mark's family, something was wrong. Mark's sister, Pauline, and our sister-in-law, Fran, looked at each other and went outside the room. My intuition, they knew Mark was in trouble. I still worked and knew I had to talk to his family but afraid to divulge Mark's secret. He'd made me swear.

On the way back to work, driving through Fresno's windy, cold valley, I thought about doing something special for Mark on Valentine's Day. He loved lobster, so I decided to steam him a live one. I enjoyed them at dinner parties before but had never cooked them. I called the grocery store and ordered two.

"Okay, Lobster Girl," I whispered in the car. "Let's give him an incredible dinner."

SECTION 2 - DOCTORS & MEMORY LOSS

On Valentine's Day, I went to pick up the lobsters. I kept my eyes on the lobster tank. It almost changed my mind. But, I promised it for dinner for Mark. It took me forever to decide which ones. Their big eyes stared at me, so difficult to pick the right ones. I apologized to the clerk for taking so long. I stood there in a trance and looked at all the lobsters. He told me to take my time. I finally pointed two in the tank. Then the butcher, who looked like the Pillsbury doughboy, put them into a wax box with air holes on top and contained with large thick rubber bands on their claws. It gave me chills to think of it. I'll never forget how difficult it was to cook them. Their eyes looked at me innocently. I picked the largest pot and filled it with water. It took me so long to throw them in, the water kept boiling down. I swore to myself never to do it again. Just the same, Mark was appreciative. He rubbed his hands together.

"Nothing better than lobster!"

A messy way to have dinner with the green gunk liver I cleaned out of the shell.

"Here's to green gunk!" Mark said in celebration of our love. He raised his wine glass to me, and I did the same. We hadn't forgotten the gravity of the situation his mother was in, but our little break from stress and uncertainty kept us going for a while. I'd sacrificed two beautiful seaworthy lobsters, and somehow, their lives gave us ours. The whole family heard about it later and had a good laugh over it.

After a few days, confronted with the need to find Mark's mom a suitable living situation, we joined in to find a skilled nursing facility. Mark, Robert, Pauline and I searched, only with disappointment. The overall environment screamed low-budget, linoleum flooring, dirty vanilla walls, shower curtains as dividers between bedroom and bathroom, worn furniture, and few caregivers among the sick residents. We observed slowly and in a visual fog, finally looking at each other in shock. Raised our eyebrows and squeezed our noses with our fingers. The unpleasant stale smell of urine and the sight of raisin shriveled bed-ridden bodies near-death was unbearable to witness. His mom needed a skilled nursing facility, but the few we checked didn't seem fit. She was in excruciating back pain, too old to have surgery, and in the transition to an assisted living, skilled nursing or a converted residential home. Painful to see what she

SECTION 2 - DOCTORS & MEMORY LOSS

went through. Yes, she was elderly and soon to be an angel in heaven, but where was the understanding of it all?

We eventually found her a small, private residential home, a conversion into an assisted living with 5 bedrooms. The residents, elderly men, and women sat in recliners, with heads drooped down asleep, stoic, lifeless, but still breathed and snored away. It smelled better and was clean, but still screamed. YOU ARE DYING!

At the facility for two days, but due to her forgetfulness and disorientation, she fell again. She went right back into the hospital. On top of the Dementia, her severe back pain was not relieved with the maximum pain meds allowed.

The next day at the hospital, his mom contracted MRSA, a staph infection. We wore gowns and masks during visiting time, to avoid any more germs brought into her room. It amazed me; they allowed us to walk in with our dirty shoes, without booties.

The doctor, the discharge nurse, and attending staff suggested that Mark's mom have an evaluation from a hospice representative. The hospital had done everything allowed to medicate her pain, but could not continue. She qualified for hospice care.

Pauline and Fran asked me to have lunch in the hospital cafeteria. I sat across from both of them in a booth. Fran started the conversation, "Jean, what's going on? Mark seems confused. Please talk to us." They were direct and looked at me in a loving and sweet way with intent and concern.

"I've wanted to talk for quite some time. Mark was adamant; I did not tell anyone." I took a deep breath, and tears rolled down my cheeks. For months, afterward, my tears seemed of their own will, separate from me, traitors and thieves, ugly scorching salty remnants of who I used to be. I never got used to it.

"Mark's diagnosis is Early Onset Dementia, the kind that turns into Alzheimer's," I said, putting down my fork. My burger sat on my plate, staring at me. French fry oil seemed thick in the air. "He doesn't want me to tell Jill and Tammy. Even though I've told him everybody loves him. They've already noticed."

"Oh, Jean, I'm going to be sick," Pauline said. "First, mom. Now, this. Horrible. Poor Mark."

Fran said, "We are sorry. We thought something was wrong. We'll be there for you."

"Thank you," I managed. "A heavy load is lifted. I know you've noticed Mark's behavior. It's been difficult hiding this." They both looked concerned and assured me of their support while holding their hands out. I told them I had to go back to the office. After I got up from the table, they both stood to hug me goodbye. My burger stayed on the table. I couldn't eat it.

In the years I knew Mark's mom, while the progression of her Dementia slowly took over, I always felt that his mom loved me for loving Mark and giving him happiness. I could see the spark in her eyes when she looked at me. Each time she greeted me, there was a look of brightness and a very tight hug.

Previously, at a family baby shower for one of the nieces, even though new to his family, his mom winked to reassure, while Mark's ex-wife sat next to his mom on purpose. I had never met the ex-wife but told she could be very charming, only to turn ice cold and ruthless. His ex-wife never gave me eye contact the entire afternoon.

His mom died a few days later in February 2008. She preferred a simple life, and her favorite thing in the last few years was spending every Tuesday lunch with her kids. The conversation and laughter made for a great time, along with the smell of fresh chocolate chip cookies for dessert. Lucky to be included in the family, I felt welcomed and a loving familiarity as my family.

At his mom's service, Mark stayed in the background. There was enough of his awareness. I imagined he didn't want anyone to ask questions, or see the stressful look on his face. In the beginning, he was embarrassed around the unwanted loss of control over his mind. He denied it. He never wanted the center of attention.

Being the executor of his mom's estate meant many financial issues to assess, address, distribute, and account for in the last six months. I stepped in without anything said to the family, but I'm sure they knew. All this

SECTION 2 - DOCTORS & MEMORY LOSS

made me more aware of my future, without Mark, financially overwhelmed. What would I do? How would I survive it?

At home, if I ran my fingers up and down the smooth grain of the wood doors that housed alarm bells, stroking the doors like willing children, could I then not slam the doors back and forth, shut and open in sheer acts of violence, letting the alarm sirens bellow across the open farmlands, fields, and streams of the valley floor? Would birds take flight? Would avalanches occur in the lower foothills from the extreme decibel levels? Who would hear it? Who would come running for me?

I loved my husband with all my heart, but unfortunately, this was a second marriage with separate assets. Could I afford to quit work before my retirement age? If I did quit, would I be able to collect disability or caregiver assistance from his social security? After his mom died, I had to make some life-changing decisions to plan for the future. Could we afford the expense of a caregiver to help out at home while I worked?

I searched the web. I tried to imagine Mark with a total stranger in the house while they prepared meals and managed our household. Would he allow it? I found out later there is no financial aid for spouses who are caregiving. In some far-off galaxy, spouses on their second or third marriage are supposed to have adequate funds and share them, not keep them separate, even for the healthiest of reasons.

I had some long, hard, exhausting thoughts about finances. I knew I had to talk to Mark at the right time.

"Will he even remember?" I asked myself over and over and out loud. "How are we going to cope financially? And oh dear Lord, how will I work full time?"

SECTION 2 - DOCTORS & MEMORY LOSS

SECTION 2 - DOCTORS & MEMORY LOSS

Chapter 9: Waiting Rooms
[2008]

After Mark's second opinion in 2008, our life resumed with all the many doctor visits. We sat in waiting rooms and I observed. I often wondered how these patients, some with elderly spouses and some alone, handled these difficult situations. Whether alone or with a spouse, they might be inexperienced with the things we tried to do. Part of me wanted to reach out to them-the decent side of me. And part of me wanted to go off on them, start a firestorm of ridiculous and crude questions I understood no one had answers to, for Mark and I or anyone in the room. My internal terrorist, something I hadn't expected to rear inside me, did without pause, and the hurricane of rage engulfed my body and kidnapped all sensibilities I previously valued, took me by complete and total shock.

A barrage of mind-chatter boxed and collided into horrific jokes in my saturated brain:

Along came the dreadfully ugly jokes: 'When I told the doctor about my memory loss, he made me pay in advance!'

In the waiting room, I shook my head hard, cleared out the cobwebs. I got down to the business to find my emotional strength in an underground locker room where internal terrorists had no key code to enter the safe walls of my authentic self. Every couple in the waiting room had it hard. None of us would get out of this alive, and never be the same.

Among the mental ability to handle the monitoring of medications, doctor visits, management of household and financial strains, and the driving — how could anyone keep it together?

To distract myself, I took notes.

But jokes like thieves of meditative calm continued to rant as I held my breath under the onslaught:

'Did you hear the one about the elephant in the bathtub? No? I can't remember it either.'

I wrote, scratching pen on paper, faster and faster as the words flowed, and my breath returned to my body. In my focus, I wanted to help others.

SECTION 2 - DOCTORS & MEMORY LOSS

From my personal experience, I wondered what others did in similar situations. Most spouses or parents were not aware of the drain, mentally, physically, and financially, unless faced with this illness. Literature I received from the Valley Caregivers and the Alzheimer's organization indicated some individuals got this disease as early as in their 30s, 40s, and 50s. There was no exact timeline.

I thought about the episodes of discord during our courtship and breakups when Mark didn't want to remarry. What if he stuck to his guns and lived alone? Who would have been responsible for his care? His daughters who lived out of town, or his siblings in town? And where would I have been? Pictured with a tropical drink in my hand as I laughed with make-believe beach friends in Hawaii. Selfish of me. I was married to someone else.

I closed my eyes and put my trembling hand over my mouth.

After three years of being on Aricept and Namenda medications, Mark's second neurologist convinced me it would serve us to take Mark to the Alzheimer Center for a third opinion. Their panel of doctors offered consultations to prepare families involved in the future.

We drove into an office complex in Fresno, in a cul-de-sac through the entrance of a bumpy parking lot, and walked into an older building, looked like the bad taste awards of the 1970s. The office furniture consisted of stale looking oak wood chairs, covered in cloth with oatmeal, avocado green, and gold colors. I hoped the staff of doctors had more up-to-date medicine and treatment solutions. I thought it sad this office environment did not receive the funding or consideration it deserved. Or maybe the doctors didn't give a crap.

That thought sent electric shivers through my spinal column.

The friendly receptionist's rehearsed smile, sweet and alarming, asked our names and handed us paperwork to complete, and later taken into a small office, we were quizzed separately, with questions from the neuropsychologist and the neurologist. The question stuck in my mind was, "How does this make you feel?" I wanted to express: Like hell, and this shouldn't be happening to us. We are young, and he looks young, fit and healthy. We have older friends, and they don't have this! A decent part of me taken away abducted without my consent. Anger like acid coursed through my veins, which caused a tightened stomach, shaky hands, and my voice to clench.

My scalp prickled. I tried to get deep, full breaths in the musty relic of the antique furniture waiting room. After this meeting, a notice will be sent to us to set an appointment to go over their findings.

In October 2008, Mark and I practically ran out to the parking lot. My wishful gaze grabbing onto anything beautiful, his face, a tired oak tree with limbs like steel girders, the aura around our faithful tan Honda Pilot, the SUV had taken us to hell and back again, sat faithfully waiting for our return. We opened the car doors and fell into our seats.

"I hate this," I said openly.

"I hate putting you through this," Mark said, scratching his forehead.

"I want to pound the steering wheel."

"Go ahead," he said. "The Pilot can take it."

I did.

The day we returned, a blustery, rainy day without ample care for getting our clothes wet or the Pilot, washed the day before, Mark's daughter Jill joined us in the parking lot.

The tension between us-Jill had not been keen on our marriage-we barely said anything. She hugged her dad. My gut lurched, led into a vanilla-looking conference room without any windows, with a rectangular table, chairs, and a few boxes of Kleenex on each side.

The neuropsychologist, an older woman with veiled green eyes and short, dark hair, introduced herself and offered us water.

"Excuse me," she said as we sat down at the table.

Staff came in and introductions were made. The neurologist, neuropsychologist, geriatrician, Jill, Mark and I were in attendance. Mark's youngest daughter, Tammy, unable to attend, but included in a conference call.

The doctor exchanged pleasantries and said, "Based on our tests and MRI, we concur with previous findings from your other physicians. Mark's frontal lobe with the most concentration of plaque, indicating Dementia, is the kind that turns into Alzheimer's disease."

I sat in the chair, practically reeling with panic. My voice came out calm. "What is the timeline of this disease?"

SECTION 2 - DOCTORS & MEMORY LOSS

"We can't estimate. The illness takes on different behaviors randomly. It typically lasts for ten years before death, depending on the onset of the illness, and it's very difficult to ascertain. There is no cure. The medication slows it down. By law, the center notifies the DMV of Mark's illness. Subsequently, DMV requests another driving test for Mark because of the findings." The doctor's veiled green eyes never flinched.

Mark looked down at the table and asked to use the restroom. He left with his head down and expressionless. It killed him. My sweet, precious loving husband was a rugged cowboy without a horse or ranch, a traveler, and drifter without a four-wheel to navigate and explore all things savage green and wild.

He won't drive again. After I heard those words, my head ballooned with pressure, as if a cloth tied to my head, choked my thoughts with disbelief. My eyes watered, and I tried to hold back tears when the doctor handed me a box of Kleenex without speaking.

While Mark was escorted, the doctor suggested an evaluation of our home by an occupational therapist, suggesting safety bars in the bath areas and an overall assessment.

"You're also going to need a Zen style home."

"Excuse me?"

"Simple. Open. Easy to maneuver."

"Zen. Do you know what Zen is?"

Every wild cat kill instinct within me wanted to launch across the table. "Yes," I said with clenched teeth. My eyes betrayed me, watering and threatening to spill over as if I were the stupidest bitch on the planet. Zen? Do you know what Zen is? I'd been a real estate specialist for over a decade. I used to meditate every Sunday afternoon. The word Zen kept going around and around like the speediest fire-tipped Ferris wheel inside my head. Good suggestions, but I was over-sensitive.

She continued. "You'll need an alarm system; bell alerts on doors to monitor Mark's activity in and out of the home. We have group support sessions in this room if you'd like to attend for counseling and education."

I listened, but numb and exhausted, while tears leaked across my cheeks and throat. I didn't want it to be real, and I prayed we'd wake up from this bad nightmare. Mark was too young. He didn't look sick. I

SECTION 2 - DOCTORS & MEMORY LOSS

prayed for mistakes. I prayed someone else's medical file was accidentally read instead of Mark's.

"Is that all?" I asked.

Jill had questions too, as did Tammy over the speaker. I pushed away from the table. What were we going to do? I couldn't live without Mark. My words died, fell from my lips to my abdomen, and then floated away. The fire-tipped Ferris wheel would not stop. Along with the forgetfulness, Mark had other previous health issues, such as his childhood asthma. He continued to cough up phlegm, so much so, I had taken him to a specialist. A previous CAT scan by a pulmonary specialist in 2003 revealed a very small dark spot on his lungs. Their diagnosis: he had Bronchiectasis, with his treatment of more inhalers. He also had chronic lower back pain. His mother had back problems, but she was in her 80's when her physical problem started.

It was my first understanding of why people shaved their heads, cut their arms, or kept twenty pill bottles near the bedside in case the longing for an overdose ached inside their secretive souls too invasively to ignore. How could I live without my Mark? How could I watch him die?

We left, and Mark was still in denial, couldn't believe it. He said, "People my age become forgetful. Nothing wrong with my driving, I've never had a ticket or been in a wreck!" His face pinched red with creases between his eyes, bruised with a look of failure, and permeated his entire being like he'd done something wrong. It was hard for him to understand. I tried to put myself in his place. Innocent and bridled, he tried to resist what would become of his future, and our future together.

"Honey, I know you are a perfect driver. This is not your fault. It's your illness. Not your fault. We don't know when it might act up and cause an accident. Someone innocent might get hurt. I love you." I hugged him and then rubbed his back. My hands brushed against the grooves of his supple and strong spine. Soon that would change. Everything would change from the loss of his memory to the loss of his health.

Envisioning him as a young boy, I attempted to trap inside my brain cells, pictures of him skipping rocks across a lake, tracking squirrels with his father, running like the wind, climbing trees and mountains hand over hand, taking on the world through the unflinching courage of his boyhood spirit. Spirits lived beyond the body. From my Catholic teachings, I grabbed onto knowledge like a shark sinking teeth: Resurrection. ... The resurrection of the body: The belief that after death, one's departed soul will be restored, or resurrected, to bodily life in heaven.

We held each other while wind swooshed more parking lot debris onto us, and Jill walked away, back to her car.

"I love you, too," Mark replied.

My sick mind went, yes, but for how long?

With a hard swallow, I followed physician advice. Our home assessed by the occupational therapist. Result-safety bars installed in the showers, alarm system installed, and with shrill bell alerts on each door to avoid possible escape without my knowledge.

Without shame, I was wondering who would ring the screaming bell on me if I left the building? If I never came back. Who, with the bell screaming for the entire neighborhood to hear, would come running after me?

I was the good-good wife, the good-good girl waiting on the rage, filtered through my bloodstream in cloying bursts, masking my acts of sanity and reason as genuine kindness. I longed to help Mark. I longed to be left alone.

"Mark, we need to organize the closest," I said briskly. Cheerful seemed necessary.

"What?"

"The closets. We need to simplify them. Mark, Zen, remember?"

He winked.

I laughed despite myself. "Zen," I said, beaming.

After I looked through the clutter of the closet in the master bedroom, I saw he never replaced things. Years went by, and so many old, different sized shirts, pants, and outdoor jackets tucked in tightly. He especially loved jackets.

"We need to put this in order," I said simply. "Throw out or give away what doesn't work right now."

"Why?" he asked. "It's my stuff. I like it."

He was resistant, and I couldn't blame him. We were shedding his things. Why couldn't we as easily shed the plaque from his brain? Instead,

I slowly boxed his old, excess clothes while he napped. A thief, I snuck his clothes out, like the internal terrorist stealing parts of him. Though exhausted and overwhelmed, I tried to keep things normal, and it was possible at times. Sure, it was. Possible. But so were frogs jumping the moon.

SECTION 2 - DOCTORS & MEMORY LOSS

SECTION 2 - DOCTORS & MEMORY LOSS

Chapter 10: Garden Talk
[2009]

It was spring in 2009, peach blossoms pink and fragrant across the valley. We always enjoyed working in the yard. Before he got sick, Mark spent many hours building a walkway of slate pavers, tucked in by Impatiens, Petunias and Zinnias, Snapdragons, and Marigolds. He loved the leveling as he kneeled, thrusting his hands to the earth, beads of sweat raining from his forehead while he worked the soil, and carefully laid the pavers, like the rocks in the foothills, the foothills we loved to hike, giving us calm and peace. The yard was our Carmel paradise, and we enjoyed working the dirt and re-working it for inspiration and possibility with each new season.

We were lucky to enjoy our backyard, the day watercolor shimmery and glistening, golden and emerald hues, bursts of neon color in reds and yellows, trees aflutter with gentle wind and birds. Mark picked this house because of the gorgeous nature of the yard, and his love for the mountains. Located near a river bottom bluff, several creatures such as foxes and raccoons lived, and many stray cats traveled from their habitat to our back yard. One early evening, we sat on our patio, enjoying a glass of wine, and Mark said, "Don't move or look behind you, there's a family of skunks walking behind you."

My skin crawled with fresh perspiration. "Shit."

While frozen in our seats, the skunks walked behind me, then in front of him, and departed from our company, as if to let us know things were different here, and they moved on to another space to live.

One particular stray, feral cat, a scrawny, calico which I grew to loathe, continued to mark its territory on our front door and screen. A wet stinking mess of cat pee, as if it was related to the internal terrorist marking my husband's territory, coating his mind with daily filth I chased the cat away with great vigor and relief, clapped my hands, shouted obscenities.

Since Mark's backache continued, I thought an above-ground planter box might serve him better. I hired a carpenter to build the large wooden planter box necessary for a vegetable garden, while he rebuilt our fence.

SECTION 2 - DOCTORS & MEMORY LOSS

We invited my dad for lunch on the patio. Mark loved my dad. Both had much in common with their artistic abilities; they loved fishing and hunting and enjoyed being outside in the garden. I served hot dogs, macaroni salad with onions, iced tea, and boysenberry pie. After small talk, I asked him, "Any suggestions on what we should add to the yard?"

"Nope. Looks good," he said. He was getting on in years, salt and pepper hair, skinnier then ever, eyes were deep brown and always happy. He missed my mom. I missed her too.

"Daddy, if you could go anywhere right now, where would you want to travel?" I asked, handing out plates of pie, with boysenberry juice all over my fingers.

He didn't answer, just contemplated. He was introspective.

My dad ended an eleven-year relationship with his live-in girlfriend. She smoked and was an alcoholic, which compounded her health problems. I couldn't understand why he was with her and supportive of those two issues; he never liked anyone who smoked or drank heavily. All I ever heard from him growing up was, "I better not catch you smoking, drinking, wearing makeup or nail polish." In my heart, he had settled and put up with her bad habits. He was 81 years old and her primary caregiver.

It was a hard transition for him, but at the same time, he knew he could no longer take care of his girlfriend. I helped my dad move out of their shared apartment and into his residence close to our home. I invited him to dinner or took him dinner frequently. He often visited us and felt comfortable enough to fall asleep before dinner on our sofa with his head hung down. He wasn't sleeping well and often woke during the night. I wanted the opportunity for one more trip with him before he couldn't travel anymore. At the same time, I knew I probably wouldn't ever be able to leave Mark alone. My heartbeat against itself with the two loves of my life.

Over the years growing up at home in Fresno, my father previously didn't know how to approach me, and couldn't communicate, so everything asked of us usually went through my mom, and his oil and acrylic or pencil drawn creations on his canvas. Before she died, she was the bearer of all news about our behavior, good or bad. He counted on her. Since she passed away, my father was better at communicating. Even though he was silent, he looked at me and smiled empathetically. He knew the impact of my situation. He saw Mark's activity in the yard, eased off from working hard to observing others' work. I discussed Mark's illness, and he was sympathetic. My dad witnessed the changes in Mark, from the slow-motion of eating, how he walked with a slight swing and limped in his gait.

Dad was in his early eighties, on a few medications, but still vital and active. I vented my frustrations to him. I got irritated when he didn't hear me. According to him, I spoke too softly. He didn't always wear his hearing aids. When I talked louder and almost yelled, he said, "I heard you." Hearing aids got tricky for us. He didn't always wear them.

In bits and pieces, like unfinished brush strokes on a white brick wall, I was losing the two most important men in my life, men who made me feel whole, valued, and loved. My husband. My Dad. Memory loss. Hearing loss. Two sides of the same coin. No one home to answer me.

Blistering obscenities at God tumbled silent and raw from my open mouth. I believed I sinned, was a sinner, woke up, and went to bed a sinner. All alarms were firing at the doors of heaven or the entrance to hell. You are being punished. You are being tortured. You are being nothing. But good.

SECTION 2 - DOCTORS & MEMORY LOSS

SECTION 2 - DOCTORS & MEMORY LOSS

Chapter 11: Family Involvement
[2010]

Friends and family did try to help. When you are a family caregiver and people hear about your suffering, wilting, deteriorating-terminal, zombie of a husband, wife, sister, brother, daughter, son, they form packs like wolves galloping mad circles around your home while howling out the latest cures for cancer, memory loss, and auto-immune disorders. Sticky notes are finger-slicked onto your front door. Try Mega Vitamin E. No signature. Left in your mailbox. Beet Juice Cures All! On your voicemail, Hey Jean. I heard Vinegar cures any memory problem. A gallon a day. Don't mind diarrhea. That's just goop squirting out. Let alone, leeches and witch spells. Blood Drains R US! Fortune Tellers crawl out of the woodwork with feverish eyes to bestow the latest remedy even if it involves a one-eyed horse and a lost herb that grows only in tar swamps. 'Seems to help....' is on every memo, e-mail, letter, text. A bad rap song...Seems-to-Seems-to-Seems-to-Hep spins without pause inside your brain cells. It becomes your parasitic mantra.

For our reasons, we stayed with our medical doctors. Was it a mistake? Looking back now, would a one-eyed horse, in a certain kind of swamp and tar dystopia, somehow have managed my husband's Alzheimer's better?

It was a routine visit to our doctor. Our normal GP. Not a specialist.

Dr. Ito of Japanese descent, middle-aged, wore wire-framed glasses and neat and calm in his white lab jacket, sat on his stool across from us in his exam room in Fresno.

"Mark," Dr. Ito addressed my husband and never wasted time or energy. Happy or sad, I believed he showed the same ceramic plate or placid lake expression. He got down to business. "Your daughter, Jill, called me."

"Called you?" Mark asked. "Why ?"

"She wants a copy of your medical records."

My heart took a hit as I slowly let out a breath in the patient's chair. His daughter hadn't cleared it with us. Was she trying to be helpful or meddling? I believed she thought we made bad medical decisions. I was seated, but it felt as if the floor was folding inward.

"Why?" I asked. The pulse in my temples thrummed.

"Her friend is a doctor. She wants him to read the test results. I told her I couldn't send copies without your permission, Mark. Violates HIPPA."

"No," Mark said instantly.

I reached for Mark's hand with his intertwined fingers. We were still a team. Mark had my back, and I had his back. Maybe innocent on Jill's part. Maybe she's trying to help. Bull, I answered. She knows what she did. Alerting, we made foolish or incompetent choices around Mark's mental health. She cut the cord and tried to take over his case. She doesn't trust me. Never did. She thought I married her dad for his money. I wanted to laugh. Mark and I sat up late many nights, talking about individual assets. How we both needed to keep them separate in case something happened. A gold digger? Yeah, that was me.

As Dr. Ito typed at his computer terminal, I pulled Mark into my shoulder. "What is Jill doing?"

"I don't know. She should have asked us."

"I feel sick."

"We're not kids, Jean. She had no right to sneak around."

"Is it possible she tried to help?"

"Help? Sure, it feels like help when someone sneaks around on you."

"She thinks we don't know what we're doing."

"Do you think we know what we're doing?"

"We're trying."

"Others will have to accept. Whether they like it or not."

"She doesn't trust me."

"But I do, Jean. That's what matters. Do you trust me?"

"I do," I said. "I always have, since we jumped out of that airplane and flew across the sky together."

In the months to come, there were suggestions from the family. Mark's brother Robert and his wife, Fran, met a local retired doctor and his wife at church. This doctor had the same illness as Mark. The wife confided she took her husband for weekly Off-Label treatments to Los Angeles, and the

SECTION 2 - DOCTORS & MEMORY LOSS

treatments seemed to help. We met the doctor, Edward and his wife, Lisa, and had dinner at their home.

Overwhelmed that afternoon, I pulled out ten different outfits, trying to decide which one made me feel the most competent. Red was too bold and aggressive. Blue too neutral and passive. It sounded like everyone said, you have no idea what you're doing. Let us help you! Let us help you, poor sad things!

Lisa, a sweet, gentle-natured woman, served store-bought deli sandwiches and salads from white cartons, and we talked openly at the dinner table like two couples getting to know each other. After dinner, her husband got up with slow and robotically stiff-jointed precision to pick up the dishes, while we helped take them to the sink. He rinsed and put them into the dishwasher. His wife invited me to look at her artwork, and we walked outside to her patio. It was the division of the sexes, men with men, women with women. Edward had similar symptoms as Mark. Yet, I didn't know how much I could take. My skin itched on my arms. I tried like hell to act courteous and friendly. Lisa was a devoted, loving wife in her eighties. As Lisa took the lead on a smooth rock pathway, the bad-rap mantra song surfaced. It felt disrespectful. I couldn't stop it from playing. Seemzto-Seemzto-Seemzto-hep.

We started our conversation at a glass-top bistro table surrounded with beautiful flowers-growing hot-house gorgeous in her garden. We both took a seat. Behind me, a miniature Meyer lemon tree stood lush and fragrant in a Japanese ceramic pot. I nearly cried from the consuming power of the bitter-sweet lemon oils.

Lisa wanted an opportunity to share away from the husbands our situations of our husbands' illnesses, without the need for a shield or mask. Our husband's diseases and behaviors were the same, but her husband was at least twenty years older (85) than Mark (65).

Mark and I crushed because we were young in comparison. Three Genie wishes in one of those moments. We'd offer up our souls for another twenty years of marriage with continued good mental health until an age-appropriate year when all could go wrong, as it was supposed to happen according to the Laws of Age and Aging. In our nineties. Not our sixties.

SECTION 2 - DOCTORS & MEMORY LOSS

I didn't wait on pleasantries. "Was Edward always like this?"

"Not in the beginning, slowly, he succumbed to it. That's why we looked for alternative treatment. It wasn't getting better. Only worse."

"Expensive?"

"Of course. FDA hasn't approved the treatments."

"Risky?"

"Well, there's always a risk, I guess. But if you mean side effects, I haven't noticed any. Mostly Edward's progress is positive. I take Edward weekly, to the clinic in southern California. If you decide to do it, maybe we can take turns driving."

I crumbled a tiny bit in the patio chair. Lisa, a beautiful eighty-year-old woman with soft gray hair cut short on her neck, bright green eyes, and a nice smile, yet behind her eyes was the look of a woman about to topple from exhaustion. How long could she keep driving Edward to southern California and not suffer from it? Caregivers suffered. I believed at that moment, quite possible, they suffered hell on earth caregiving their spouses.

"Insurance?" I asked.

"Forget it."

"Nothing?"

"Not one cent." She sighed, her smile lighting up the patio. "I wish I could say it won't drain your bank account. I wish for a lot of things."

I reached for her hand and stroked it. "Me too," I said.

A few minutes later, we went into the house. Mark and the doctor conversed as though they had not a care in the world. They both seemed perfectly normal and engaged in a nice sports exchange. The couples' small poodle kept jumping up onto the sofa to protect his master. The retired doctor didn't respond to the dog. I leaned down and started to pet the dog, and Mark joined me.

I gave a lot of thought about this experimental treatment, not clinically tested and it scared the crap out of me. Was it worth investigating and pursuing? After much discussion, Mark and I decided to meet the doctor for a consultation in southern California.

"You ready for this?" Mark asked me.

"Not at all," I said.

SECTION 2 - DOCTORS & MEMORY LOSS

"Me, either."

We drove south to the offices Lisa recommended, located near the university through the rolling hills of the campus, and checked into the bungalows for rent. The next day, we sat in the waiting room at the doctor's office and asked to complete a questionnaire, along with submitting a consultation fee of $350. We consulted with Dr. Greg Jones and saw the equipment used for treatments. If we signed up for care, the consultation fee went toward the procedure. If we bowed out, the consultation fee not reimbursed.

We watched a video of testimonials by individuals and their families of all ages and viewed different brain issue experiences. Each testimonial of patients portrayed their loved ones pitching the significant benefits to treatment and their improvements. There were young individuals with brain injuries and older patients with memory issues that stemmed from different diseases. I'll admit I was skeptical, yet hopeful. For once, the bad rap mantra-seemztohep did not play.

"What do you think?" I asked Mark.

"Let's do it," he said.

Focusing on the shooting light of hope in his eyes, I agreed. I'd gotten so used to his deadeyes. It was something. Anything. It was exactly what we needed the most: purpose.

After signing many forms, we went into the reception area and waited for the consultation. After introductions, we followed Dr. Jones, a dermatologist, into his office. Not a neurologist?

"Dermatology?" Mark asked. "I don't understand."

Dr. Jones smiled, his charisma like an aura glowing inside the room. "Let me explain."

We sat in chairs. I felt frozen. How does this dermatologist think he can suggest treatment for my husband's brain? Dr. Jones jumped in. "The drug of treatment is administered in the neck. Then the patient stands in front of a vertical gurney and is strapped on tight. With the head upright, the body is turned upside down, so their head faces toward the floor. Let's go into the exam room so I can show you." Both speechless at this point, but in my mind, QUACK barreled over my rational thoughts. Mark looked at me skeptically. Vulnerable to the situation and lived in a time of such uncertainty, we might have tried any new remedy. How do I respond to this? Stay? Run?

Dr. Jones finished. "Any questions?"

"Thank you, doctor, we need to go home and think this over," I said. I don't need to think this over, it's wrong. We left, and I tried to compose myself.

"Mark, I won't put you through that," I said after we were in the car.

"I agree. Let's go home." He looked at me with a sense of relief and smiled. "Jean, I love you so much."

"I love you too."

"What now?"

"I have no idea."

Weeks later, we contacted the medical staff from San Francisco clinical trials for patients like Mark with memory loss, even though through the university, there were no assurances Mark would get the treatment, the risk, that he might get the placebo. We discussed a possibility but decided not to try. We didn't want to attempt the frequent drives to San Francisco with no guarantees.

We resumed our unpredictable life. Mark diagnosed, and his daughters, brother, and sister were informed. We did the best we could, in the new normal of the uncertain game of Memory Loss Monopoly. Almost every step we took for real and lasting help or care brought us back to the start. Do not pass 'Go.'

* * *

During this time, Mark's daughter Jill married. We dealt with family dynamics, especially with Mark's ex-wife, Lucy. Conflict arose between Jill and her mother over the number of friends attending, and Jill said, "Dad, I don't know how you lived with her for so long."

His daughter's wedding was a stressful event for Mark to maneuver.

SECTION 2 - DOCTORS & MEMORY LOSS

He was guarded, disoriented, and off-balance in a different place. He escorted his daughter down steep winding stairs from the bluff clubhouse, down to the golf course lawn to the aisle to give his daughter away. I was in constant watch of him. Aware of his illness, everyone was curious about his condition and paid attention to him. He was particularly noticeable in his tux and baseball hat, adorned to keep his head from sunburn.

Somehow, he made it. He even posed for pictures taken throughout the evening. He danced with his daughter while he wore a crown fashioned from a tie wrapped at his forehead, which his favorite niece created. Missed was his voice to say thank you to the family and friends, and the toast to his daughter and new son-in-law. Still, he wore a continual smile and showed his happiness for his daughter. He got through it, even though he was in the mid to late stages of the disease, and it overwhelmed him to engage in a setting in front of a crowd.

* * *

Months later, at home, Mark walked in the bedroom, with a feverish-red look of stress on his face. A conversation with Jill hadn't gone well. Agitated, he said, "Jill called, and she needs money. She wants to know how much money I have." He looked at me with raised eyebrows.

Angry butterflies filled my stomach. I wasn't calm. Between the two of us, hashing out our dilemma, I thought we might do more damage than good. "Can we talk about this later?" I asked.

"O.K."

I didn't know what to do, except wait until we calmed down.

Later I talked to Mark. I knew the talk with his daughter would be difficult, always a rub because of the ex-wife, Lucy, and her influence over of his daughters, Jill and Tammy.

His brother and I were both the successor co-trustees of his estate. Mark always told me he never wanted to reveal to his daughters his worth. He didn't want his ex-wife to know his business.

SECTION 2 - DOCTORS & MEMORY LOSS

"Mark, do you want me to call Jill and talk to her?" I asked.

"Yes," he said.

"Do you want to relieve yourself of the pressure of the estate? Maybe pass the succession to your brother and me?" I hesitantly asked.

"Yes," he replied.

I assumed Mark told his daughters that his brother and I were successor co-trustees of his estate. Angry Jill didn't trust me enough to talk. I made the phone call.

"Hello, Jill. It's Jean." Mark listened and watched as I spoke.

"I didn't call him because I needed money," Jill said to me.

"Well, I think there was a miscommunication. Your dad thought you needed some money. Your dad made your uncle and I co-trustees of his estate. I assumed you knew. Don't worry about your dad's estate. I don't have sole access to your father's money, both your uncle and I are co-trustees. We both have to sign on any matter."

"Don't take this personally, but I thought my sister and I were co-trustees. I didn't know there were any changes or would be any changes. I just wanted to find out if my dad has enough money for his care."

After the conversation, I understood I needed to contact Mark's doctor and document everything regarding his care and the estate's trust for Mark. I called Mark's trust attorney to get advice from him, and counseling advice from the neuropsychologist at the Alzheimer's Center. I scheduled an appointment, and during that session, I told her of the family dynamics of a second marriage with adult children. The doctor assured me I handled all of the affairs the right way. Regarding his health, since I'm his primary on his Health Care Directive Order, his health decisions ultimately were my responsibility. I was the one caring for him should the bottom fall out.

Even so, I knew, in my heart, I would always talk over all of Mark's health with his brother and sister, who were local. They made themselves available to help support me. And I would keep his daughters informed on his status.

Needing space in a big way, I told Mark I was going outside for a few minutes. I looked at everything in our modest home and walked out into our backyard and took some deep breaths. I recalled a question Mark asked me weeks before we got married, "Do you want to move into my house, or do you want to buy a bigger house?"

"No, let's stay here. I don't want anything bigger."

I was glad I'd made that decision. I didn't want the extra burden of the financial responsibility for a larger house.

SECTION 2 - DOCTORS & MEMORY LOSS

SECTION 2 - DOCTORS & MEMORY LOSS

Chapter 12: Hallway
[2010]

Early evening we watched TV in 2010. Mark sat next to me on our love seat, while he stared off in another direction with a pale and stoic look. At times I intermittently looked at him and journaled my tablet of our daily events. He went into the kitchen at least three times and brought three glasses of water by his side. I stopped asking why he needed so much water. I finally accepted he got the water for the people he saw while controlled by the internal terrorist. I often thought of what other repetitive actions or behaviors would ensue in our lives together. The water was simple.

After the educational courses, I learned how to cope with Mark's symptoms, and I tried to be more patient and less anal about things. I hired a housekeeper weekly instead of twice a month. I was less of a cook and more of a take-out queen of white cartons, serving frozen TV dinners and store-bought deli sandwiches. I was more of an observer.

Gardening was my greatest elixir. I hoped Mark came along, but he lasted 5 or 10 minutes. He wanted to hoard and hide things inside. In keeping with the goals of his internal terrorist illness, our precious things went missing, my rings in the garbage. His money tucked into folds of Saran Wrap. Re-ordered printed checks from the bank.

The complete and total invasion of his body and mind changed his independent nature, causing him to become beyond needy and clingy with me. I learned to accept the ups and downs but desperately wished for a miracle. What I understood as my constant, I loved my Mark more deeply every day. Yes, I got to spend more time with him, but he slowly slipped away. He became paranoid, thinking the housekeeper or a stranger stole his things.

I thought he needed a change of scenery. So, I planned a trip before Christmas to see his daughters and take Christmas gifts. I invited his brother and sister-in-law to stay with us in our timeshare. It was a long-distance, but fun for him to see his kids and grandchildren, and spend time with his brother and sister-in-law.

SECTION 2 - DOCTORS & MEMORY LOSS

We had such a great time, we thought of taking another trip, maybe a cruise to Alaska. It seemed like such a good idea, and no one would have to drive. Easy for Mark. Easier on me. Nice to fantasize about it.

Even though his out-of-town daughters were not much help, they made suggestions by phone. Jill knew of a wellness clinic and highly recommended it. After discussing it with the clinic's program director, I discussed it with Mark. It meant a trip to southern California for a week, possibly two.

Nothing on the clinic's website indicated any success with Dementia or Alzheimer's patients. Still I leaned toward taking him for a consultation because of Mark's other issues with allergies and asthma. Nevertheless, I had to give it a try, knowing if I didn't, his daughters would say, 'she didn't try.' Is this a waste of time and money?

Plus, my hope was sorely in question. I hated being negative ninety-percent of the time. I'd never been this negative in my life. It wasn't me.

The clinic was costly; plus, I needed to be with Mark at all the sessions. I had to watch him. He couldn't be left alone. I talked to my boss about the time off, and he understood and said, "Do what's best for your family."

In addition to the wellness clinic trip, I added a mini-vacation, a short 2-day road trip, one night at the central coast, and another near Santa Barbara. I realized it might be a long trip, with too many changes, but took the chance. I wanted a fun trip for Mark with a change of scenery, and hopefully, to enjoy it. I told him it was for our tenth anniversary.

"We're going to have the best time!" I said, driving the car down Highway 99 south. Mark, fastened into the passenger seat, didn't answer me.

I chose an older beautiful boutique hotel with Spanish hacienda architecture in Montecito, California. The grounds had a lush landscape, aromatic lavender, organic gardens, and lily ponds. Each cottage suite was romantically decorated with fireplaces, cut fresh flowers, fresh fruit, chocolate truffles, wine, and a flowered patio, with a bistro table and chairs to enjoy it all. We hiked, as we always loved nature and the outdoors. He seemed to enjoy those two days genuinely; in fact, we both did. It was an extravagant trip for our budget, but I thought it might be our last trip.

SECTION 2 - DOCTORS & MEMORY LOSS

On the drive to the wellness clinic, we reminisced of his marriage proposal to me.

"Mark, I can't believe it. It's been ten years."

"What?"

"Remember the margaritas you poured. My proposal. Especially my ring."

"Oh, yeah. Sure do."

"The one you made. Twisted-knot napkin ring. You put an ice cube on top. For a mock-diamond."

"Really?"

"I loved it! Especially the note you wrote. Dated May 22, 2000, you said, 'I want you to be my wife. In this lifetime.'"

* * *

Deterioration on all earthly planes, mental, physical, spiritual, happened rapidly after some months for Mark. For me, it was slower, my changes like tar sludge surging up and down my veins instead of blood. All battered like old ropes on a dock savaged by wind and rain and salt, yet, I had to try. We had to try; alternative clinics, faith healers, tricksters, and snake oil salesmen all lined up to scoop out our pains and slide our last dollar through the credit card machines.

In the middle of the night, I jerked awake. Pound-pound-pound! Where was I? Pound-pound-pound. Throwing off the coverlet of the bed, I blinked in utter darkness, swooned with panic as my hand grasped space, and I fumbled for the lamp on the bed stand. Pound-pound-pound. "Just a minute." I got the switch. Light bathed the room. Blinking-blinking, as I jumped out of bed. God help me here. Okay. Hotel room. Newport Beach, California. "Who's there?" I yelled.

A woman's voice, "THE HOTEL NIGHT MANAGER. OPEN UP."

What could this be? I opened the door to find Mark standing in his pajamas. His head drooped as he stood next to the night manager. There was no recognition on his white-plated face, minor shadows flitting across his cheeks and chin from outside, and no understanding of where he was or-gulp-what he did. My throat squeezed shut even though my mouth was open. Air hissed through my upper teeth. Oh, dear God, how did this happen? How did he get out of the room without me hearing him leave?

"I tried to call you. No answer," the manager said.

How did I not hear that phone?

"Excuse me," I said, while I put my arms around Mark and helped him in. His pajama bottoms soaked in a strong scent of urine. I walked back to the door. The woman manager wrinkled her nose, and leaned toward my ear, whispered my husband wandered in the halls, and peed all over the floor.

"What?"

"He peed. The hall floors."

"Oh God, Did anyone…?"

"We got a call."

"We're any children…saw him and…?"

"Oh no. Nothing like that. It's late. "

"Police?"

"Not that I know of."

Adrenaline shot through me like lit gasoline. The muscles in my upper back twitched with anger. I stayed stoic, acting in control as a countermeasure to my husband's incredulous urine mess outside. In my heart, I was seething, my palms and fingertips shaking involuntarily at Mark's outrageous and dangerous behavior, even if he was disoriented. I pressed palms and fingers into my hips to prevent shaking. The cops could have been called!

"He must have mistaken the entrance door as the bathroom door. I'm so very…."

"You need to barricade the door."

"What?"

"Keep him from coming out again."

"Yes." I dug my toes into the rug. "Can I please call you in the morning?"

"No need."

"But his Dementia…I need to let you know about…"

"People stay here. For the health clinic. Often."After she left, huffing with red-faced embarrassment and fatigue, I shoved and pushed to build a luggage barricade against the front door.

SECTION 2 - DOCTORS & MEMORY LOSS

A firestorm of apocalyptic thoughts assailed me. What if Mark walked into the abyss of the city, lost wandering the streets, and crossing heavy traffic.

The next afternoon, I bought tiny bells and slivered ribbons to tie together and hung from the doorknob, pretty decorations for the ugliest of reasons. Not only Mark's wife, but I also became his warden.

From the luggage-walled and fortified confines of our hotel room to the entombed fluorescent-lit ceiling of the alternative wellness clinic in Newport Beach, we walked hand in hand to the reception, greeted with joviality and instructions from the staff. Around fifty couples appeared decades older than Mark or I. Why did it matter? Because it did. Even after spending a half-hour in the shower, I wasn't able to grasp the reality, still scrubbing off any traces of Mark's urine, from me. Scrubbing-scrubbing, even though none remained on our skin. We were too young. This was all a mistake. Screaming seemed the hands-down more appropriate response over the socialized exchange of grins and niceties. As if in making the exact right choice, we somehow won the lottery of good mental health.

Hating myself, split between forgiving Mark or my irritation, my slap-stick mind cut loose on a stage of sarcasm and focused on what they would serve us at the banquet. Not shit white flour rolls. I hate those rolls!

"Let's go into the banquet room, dinner will be served soon," the staff cooed.

We all shuffled in like cows to the riverbank, plunked down in padded seats at round tables.

The doctor came in, a squat, beaming man in his mid-forties; cropped black hair, heavily lidded eyes. "Hello, hello," he said. "My name is Dr. Sandford. Welcome to our fabulous clinic."

I sighed, felt spent to my fingernails and let down, it was pathetic. I kept putting my cloth napkin in my lap, picking it up again, folding it on the table. Then smoothed it across my thighs. Picked it up. Catering staff appeared and brought in leafy salads. Mark barely flinched, his face surreal and nearly cardboard. Little bolts of pain zinged my throat. I ached to say to Mark, "And if you liked that one, did you hear the one about the mule at the bar?"

SECTION 2 - DOCTORS & MEMORY LOSS

Dr. Sandford continued. "Many of you have traveled a vast distance to be here with us tonight. I applaud those of you who have come by airplane, bus, train, or car." All that I could think is, 'See Jane run. Watch Jane drive.'

Trapped in alternative wellness-land, I wasn't doing well. I assumed all attendees at the banquet wished for a sudden electric explosion of fireworks and magic, a futuristic display of newly cloned life bred for extraction of healthy brains and organs, like the plot in the movie, The Island.

"Does anyone have any questions before we start eating?" he asked.

What the hell was I supposed to ask? I thought about injecting this banquet room with verbal suicide. What happened to us? Why is my husband losing his mind?

To my complete shock, not one question asked. Blind trust was the shits.

After dinner, we tried to sleep early in our hotel room. I looked at the clinic's first day's schedule of the rigorous barrage of treatments and prayed Mark was able to handle. I didn't know what to expect. I tossed and turned that night in our hotel bed, sweating, hands shaking, stomach clutching, tried to sleep even as I thought Mark might get out again. Clanging metal chains with shackles seemed in order, wrapping his neck to feet looked in order. If he got out and peed again in the hallway, I could succinctly hear the cops at our hotel door, 'Ma'am. You let him out? What's wrong with you? Yes, he took a catwalk near the swimming pool to pee. Of course, you're under arrest.'

The next morning the clinic blood was drawn with results given by a red-headed female, alternative-health doctor. We sat in a boxy office with Mark's adult daughter Jill. Jill was as anxious as we were. She cared for and loved her dad. With her beautiful brown hair and huge eyes, she sat in the corner next to us, as dumb-founded, concerned, and unnerved as we were.

"Mark's questionnaire indicates fatigue, fuzzy thinking, muscle weakness, and joint pain. His saliva test indicates a yeast infection caused by Candida. I'm prescribing medication for it and advise you to read a book that details foods in your diet, which exacerbate the problem." She pen-scratched in Mark's patient file. "There will be supplements, of course. Tons. You might have to crush them."

"Supplements?"

"Herbals. Vitamins. Good stuff."

SECTION 2 - DOCTORS & MEMORY LOSS

She checked Mark's file. "How did you hear about us?"

"What?" I asked.

"How were you referred?"

"Uh, Mark's daughter, Jill."

"I read about the clinic in a magazine," Jill added.

The doctor scribbled more. Mark and I looked at each other.

"There's a couple more things. Part of his program includes detoxification medications to remove heavy metals found in his blood. And his testosterone is low, so hormone enhancements are prescribed." Mark looked at me for an answer. I lifted my eyebrows. What was I supposed to say? He can't find the bathroom from a hole in the ground, but hey...I'll be sure he knows which pill to take.

"Dad, mom had heavy metals in her blood too." Mark didn't respond.

"You know," the doctor said. "I'm not even sure he has Dementia."

"Excuse me," I said.

"What?" Jill asked.

"Nope. Not sure." We're paying you to be sure.

"Not sure at all." She finished with the file and snapped it shut.

She's not a neurologist. How does she think she's qualified to say that? My first red flag went up.

Day One of Treatment - Shuttled to the clinic, missed hotel 7:00 a.m. breakfast. The scene at the clinic looked like a horror movie - Enter a room, sign in on a clipboard. Fragile patients, including my husband, hooked to I. V. drips. Tie, rub, stab, repeat. Breakfast delivered while Mark's I. V. drip insect cocoon hung along with twenty other IV bottles row by row. Hungry? Blood transfusions, drip-drip-drip. Unbelievable. Four hours went by. Too slow to live through. All the family and spousal caregivers want to jump from a window.

As I shadowed Mark, I observed I was one of few spouses or partners with their significant others. Surprised to see a famous actor who received a treatment, and walked over and introduced himself, as if we didn't recognize him.

Next, the Hyperbaric Oxygen chamber room with machinery positioned above the floor and was like the cockpit of a wingless airplane. Inside at the front, a video played while Mark watched scenes

SECTION 2 - DOCTORS & MEMORY LOSS

and listened to music. The compressed hundred percent of oxygen trapped him, like a caged rat bombed with repellent. Sorry, all this to maybe help his brain. I can't help it, but this makes my skin itch.

"Why don't you do this, Jean?" He was claustrophobic.

"No, this is special for you. It looks like a fun ride, but too expensive for both of us. I'll sit outside and face you." I moved a chair outside and sat next to him.

"You can wave your hand at the window for anything you need. I'll be right here." He shook his head. The attendant explained the experience to him. I sat as if happy. I hoped he wouldn't see through my phony smile, the one I wore nearly 24/7 like the white bone base of an artifact on display.

He waved to me, wincing, moaning. His ears popping, he lasted a half hour. I didn't blame him.

Last ride for the day, an EEG Analysis for the Neuro-map of Mark's brain. Our attendant, an olive-skinned young man, especially sympathetic, said, "I know this is hard on both of you, but we'll get you through it."

He asked Mark to sit in front of a computer monitor, and he placed several rounded, flat electrodes on his head and forehead. The wires connected from his head to machinery and hooked up to the computer. This test monitored his brain waves on things he saw or heard through the earphones. He explained each action slowly to accommodate our particular situation. This does feel like science fiction. I can't believe he's not trying to take the machinery off. It must be good music with the movie. This was a grueling first day. My mind absorption competed with my middle finger callus, which grew faster as I journaled everything and also wanted to stick it up in the air.

The same evening, a Sleep Apnea test kit was given to me to administer on Mark. The equipment wrapped around his forehead, the sides of his face and onto his nose. During the night he was supposed to wear it and kept taking it off. I couldn't blame him. I unhooked it.

"The hell with this," I said to him. "It's too much. I should have known."

"Know what, Jean?"

"We're in a maze of revolving doors."

SECTION 2 - DOCTORS & MEMORY LOSS

"Like Disneyland?"

"No. More like gothic horror. Doctor Jekyll and Mr. Hyde."

While at the clinic, day in and day out, both his daughters tried to relieve me. Mark's oldest daughter came one afternoon during his session on the EEC table, and he used a non-invasive treatment used to lower the risk of angina episodes. Jill, a striking brunette with long legs, walked out to make a phone call and told him she would be right back. He unstrapped himself and walked outside to look for her. This was not her dad, he was like a forgetful child lost at camp. His memory and decision-making did not allow him to be alone in this environment unattended. He was vulnerable away from home in this strange setting.

Mark's youngest daughter, Tammy, called the day after and said she wanted to relieve me for an hour and a half, in between classes during the week. I declined and said, "I know you mean well, but an hour and a half won't help me. Why don't you just visit him?" I'm sure she thought I was a bitch, but I couldn't leave him. Even though I believed her offer to help was sincere, it was a drop of sand in an hourglass with nothing leftover but air to grasp.

Back at the hotel on Saturday after a day of treatments, I looked at the clinic's outlined chart for prescriptions and supplements. I laid the pills and a glass of water on the table and pointed at them. Mark's sour look did not help matters.

"Mark, evening pills." He went next to the table.

"No more pills," he whined.

Pills fell on the floor, and my blood pressure skyrocketed to a million. My head began to split. If I didn't do something fast, it wouldn't be pretty inside our hotel room prison cell. Death and mayhem, blood, and guts. The warden due to her one-hour break.

"I'm calling Tammy. We need time apart."

He rolled his eyes. "Oh, brother!" Now, where did I put those chains and shackles?

It was Saturday, and we'd both had enough. We had been through the treatments for at least ten days. I telephoned his children to please pick him up. As soon as they left, I showered and went to the store to buy a few things. I wasn't sure of the lay of the land, but I went downstairs and asked

SECTION 2 - DOCTORS & MEMORY LOSS

the concierge for help. I walked into the grocery store to buy a few snacks for the room and walked up and down the aisles. I couldn't figure out what I wanted. Not hungry at the time, I ended up buying string cheese, apples, crackers, and water. The distraction was what I needed, an escape from reality for just a little while.

That evening I received an unexpected call from my father. He said, "I'm just checking in to see how everything is going."

"It's hard, the days are long with all of his treatments," I said.

"I was just thinking about you. I love you." Wow. I'd always had to say it to him first.

"I love you too, daddy," I said, sinking into the bed like a found rag doll.

SECTION 2 - DOCTORS & MEMORY LOSS

Chapter 13: Dad
[2010]

Back at the clinic, I sat in the waiting room and kept my distance, while Mark had a treatment to give ourselves space. We hadn't quite recovered from our argument over his pills. The woman next to me appeared calm and friendly and I needed both, even if she was a stranger. I left messages for my dad, and either he hadn't received them, or something happened, and he wasn't able to call. Our calls usually instantaneous, he called and left a message, and I called him right back. Rare for us to skip hours without bugging each other.

"Hi," I said to her. "I'm Jean. How's it going?"

"Good. It's a good day for my husband and me."

"Not so good for us. We fought last night. Stupid pills."

"Oh, yes. The pills. You'd think we made them down some poison."

I laughed. She was nice and her name was Lisa. I blew out a long slow breath. "I usually talk to my dad every day. He's my support buddy. I can't reach him. When I get a hold of him, I'm gonna yell. I hope he's with a new friend, and just hasn't called me."

"You mean a girlfriend?"

"Well, my mom died some years ago. She was hit by a car while walking on a street."

"That's terrible."

"Yes, it was." I felt suddenly flush with shame, almost too selfish with the disclosure of how my mom passed away. It wasn't Lisa's fault. She had troubles of her own to dog-paddle through if she was here at the clinic.

To recover, I asked, "How are things going for you?"

"I've been better," she replied. She smiled sympathetically, preoccupied with her thoughts.

I decided to leave her alone. It was June 9, 2010, and Mark and I were at the clinic for eleven days until the next day and another attempt to reach my dad was unsuccessful. I called Ann. She was my rock when all else failed.

SECTION 2 - DOCTORS & MEMORY LOSS

"Ann, will you please drive to grandpa's apartment? See if his car is parked outside."

"I'm out right now. I will go in a half-hour." She said

"Thanks, sweetheart."

She called in forty minutes. "Mom, I drove by. I didn't see his car." Where can he be?

"Ann, I'll call his apartment manager and beg them to please break in to check. Claw scratches of terror raced across my chest. I had an ache in my neck gripped my skull, and a nagging thought wouldn't stop. Please no. Not my dad. All I could do was wait to find out.

An hour later, we had a consultation with the clinic's nutritionist.

Lastly, we were in the EEG Analysis, and Mark had electrodes on his head. My head spun like a revolving door. To distract myself, I monitored treatments and took notes. At the same time, I tried to reach my Dad again and couldn't. Then a phone call came in. I motioned to the-attendant I would be right back, and left Mark still hooked to the machinery. I answered the phone call from a man who introduced himself as a Police Officer. Terrified, I walked outside of the building, the sunlight outside shifting in my vision. In case I fell, I looked for the first car in the parking lot to hold me.

"Is this Jean?" he said calmly.

"Yes," I replied.

"We found your dad on the floor of his apartment. He's still breathing, but unconscious. What hospital would you like us to take him to?"

It felt as though a million needles were in my head. My eyes blurred and cleared. Then, I came to my senses and said, "My father is a World War II vet, he goes to the V. A., but please take him to the closest hospital, St. Agnes."

"We're on our way," he said.

What do I do? The parking lot spun, raced away from me, slowed down, and my feet like lead. I can't seem to put anything in order. We are five hours away. We need to leave. Call Ann.

"Ann, the police broke into grandpa's apartment. He was on the floor, still breathing. They're taking him to St. Agnes. I'm coming home."

SECTION 2 - DOCTORS & MEMORY LOSS

I stood outside of the building, tried to figure it out. Get a grip. You need to organize. Get home safe. How will I drive us back five hours and hold it together? What about Mark? We're cutting his treatment short. No other option.

Ann's sobs filled the phone.

"Mom, I drove by and didn't see his car."

I took a deep breath, turning in a circle of invisible glue. "Ann, pull over and park, his new car was there. I think you might have been looking for his old car."

"Mom, how are you so calm?" Ann's weeping escalated.

I remembered her as a child when she learned to ride her bike. She couldn't brake and ran into her dad's bike. How she bawled and bawled and said, "Mommy, I hate days like today."

"I love you, honey," I said. My thoughts swung from panic to gratitude. So thankful Ann didn't see her grandfather that way.

I called a good friend to be with Ann at the hospital until I got home. As soon as I knew Ann was okay, I called Mark's daughters. Then I started to sift through the best plan to get home, as soon as possible. I learned many things at the beginning of this journey with Mark's illness. Plans made evaporated in seconds, reconstructed and torn down, like printed words pulled off an Etch a Sketch or a Magic White Board. I walked to the wellness facility manager and told her we had to leave.

The shuttle ride back to the hotel was long. I looked out the window. I can't tell you what I saw. At that moment, I couldn't help but think: Could I trust myself to drive both Mark and myself back?

Until I received a call from Mark's new son-in-law, who offered to drive us the five hours to Fresno, then I notified the hotel management of our emergency. Total chaos with clothes, shoes, and medications strewn inside the hotel room.

"We have to pack, now Mark. Right, this minute. Throw everything in the suitcases." I said.

Mark floated in and out of knowing there was an urgency of matters to maneuver. He kept saying, "Now what are we doing? Now, what are we doing?"

"We're going home," I said every time.

SECTION 2 - DOCTORS & MEMORY LOSS

The drive home was emotional, reflective, and haunting. Sorry, my daughter had to pitch in, knowing in my heart, it was very serious. I tried not to think of my dad and how long he was in that state, frozen or hurt on the floor of his apartment, conscious or not, unable to move.

The last time he came to dinner at our house in Fresno. I walked outside with him and hugged him, told him I loved him and watched him slowly walk to the car. I remember thinking, His walk is different. How long will he be able to drive here and come to dinner? He was the dad who always called me, rain, shine, sleet, hail, on into the night of no return for any of us. Dad! Dad! Dad! Please don't go.

* * *

I remembered a time as a young girl, thinking as a young girl prone to fits of black imagination, that my loving father died. One evening, I opened the front door to see my father crying and kneeling on the ground, with blood dripping from his head as if a faucet of bloody water drained from his skull. The porch light shined behind his head like a halo. He was out with friends when attacked by a mugger, who knifed him on his temple. Everyone shocked how he was able to drive home that night. I remember my mother spooning sugar in my mouth from the shock of it all. He was hospitalized. I couldn't get it out of my mind how my dad looked, and I thought he died because he wouldn't come home. At that time, children weren't allowed to visit inside the hospital, but I was finally taken outside his hospital room. I stood outside by his window, heard his voice and said hello. It gave me comfort to know my dad was healing when I heard his voice. He was a strong warrior, but it pressed hard on my mind.

* * *

In so many ways, my dad's tenderness was akin to Mark's. Mark often would rub my leg to help me fall asleep. As a child, my dad always made sure to fan my brother and me to sleep, when our house in the country was warm. He made sure we were bundled in warmth if it was cold. It didn't matter what I thought about around my dad, our childhood, or what just

SECTION 2 - DOCTORS & MEMORY LOSS

happened to him; it all made me cry. This was the longest drive of my life. I decided to call my daughter again to see if my father's CT scans came back. And they had.

"Mom, the doctor said grandpa had a severe stroke. They have him on a ventilator. We need to make a decision. We can do surgery, but there's no guarantee. The doctor said, 'If it was my dad, I wouldn't do the surgery.' Mom, you need to decide what to do. Once you do, there's no going back. They'll keep him on the ventilator till you let me know."

Empty, no one home inside me. "Let me call you later," I said.

I knew my father didn't want any heroics, but at the same time, how could I make this decision? In my heart, I knew my father was never the same after my mom died. Did he give up? Should I let him go to Heaven and not put him through the surgery?

All this internal drama played in my head, while Mark and his son-in-law sat in the front seat and carried a normal conversation. I picked up my cell for the horrific call.

"Ann, please keep grandpa on the ventilator until I get there." I wept almost the entire trip to the hospital.

Mark's son-in-law dropped me off at the hospital. They went home. I walked into the barely lit room and immediately hugged my daughter and son-in-law. They had heavy bags under their eyes. I went to my father and hugged him, told him I loved him, and wept some more. How much water do our bodies have to keep crying? I touched his face, and it felt warm. Then, I lifted the blanket carefully, which covered my father and touched his fingers. They felt very cold. Is this what death feels like? My strong warrior, my dad, who always wanted to protect my family and me. He looked so vulnerable and peaceful at the same time. He was in transition. Take me with you, I thought for a brief second. Knowing it was wrong. Knowing I loved my husband, my daughter, son-in-law and grandkids. Knowing I had to pull the plug.

* * *

My father, though not tall, was strong and mighty in many ways, and full of wisdom. He was a World War II Veteran warrior at seventeen years

SECTION 2 - DOCTORS & MEMORY LOSS

old. He traveled with the Navy on the USS Missouri, where the peace treaty was signed on September 2, 1945. He hardly spoke about the war but loved opening a file tin box of black and white pictures of him and his buddies, all dressed in uniform, along with all the other naval officers on the second tier, intently watching as the peace treaty was signed.

He observed ranks in the war, saw a chain of command, and that education was necessary to move up in the world.

"Always have a system," the way he told us to be organized and ambitious. He expressed his ideas, excitedly with a deep breath, licked his lips and then began our lesson. Usually, after a few drinks of cheer, he expressed it more easily and with much emotion, sometimes with tears. Those were the times we heard how much he loved us and would do anything. He was naturally artistic, quiet and gentle. Most of all, he was our rock. His heritage came from Mexico and Spain, with parents who didn't speak English. The children made fun of my dad and my uncle for their lack of English and going barefoot to school.

* * *

Conflict within my soul. Dad needed my release, mechanically, and in my heart. I had to let him go to Heaven. He would be with my mom in eternal peace. I sat there and watched him. I thought of all he accomplished. He was my hero. I would let him go. It was what was supposed to happen. So many things went through my mind. He was happy after he retired. All he wanted was to spend time with his family and his passion to draw and paint.

The hardest words I ever had to say were the words to the nurse. As I kept swallowing, my mouth and throat watered, to ask the nurse to unhook my dad's ventilator.

"Please…"

"Excuse me? What's that?"

"Please unhook…"

"What did you say?"

"…unhook…my dad's…"

"Oh. Oh, yes, I see now."

SECTION 2 - DOCTORS & MEMORY LOSS

Let him go. Let him go. And I did, following the path of her steady piano fingers, her deft routine with gears and gizmos and machines, she maneuvered with rehearsed sterility. Needles, catheters, IV bags removed with small whispers and clicks and beeps. Then deafness for me, falling through a crushing abyss of darkness, tumbling so fast the end of his death brought me to the evaporated end of my inner strength, salted wounds at the bottom of a very deep well. A fierce little girl, weep, escaped through my teeth.

The nurse didn't hear it. "So sorry," she said with her back to me, flicked off switches, unplugged cords. Somewhere between a quarter-tone of genuine caring and the exhausted tone used for tomorrow's grocery list, she swung in my direction and said, "Take your time." Then shoulders squared, she snatched up her supplies and with a sigh of relief hustled from the room where she left me to find my way out again.

It was June 10, 2010.

* * *

The day of the memorial service, the sun shined on the mausoleum building. Remembered as a World War II Veteran with a 21-gun salute, the older veterans faced the sun and saluted their friend, my father, with the respect due, for his dedicated service to the United States of America, risking his life in the war, and heard by the firing of the rifles in his honor. The American flag along with the caps of the bullets handed to me. His body placed at the reserved spot next to our mom, who died fourteen years before.

A luncheon held at his favorite Basque restaurant, that he'd frequented many times for dinner and music. Mark sat with his daughters at another table during the entire luncheon. He didn't understand I needed his support. Life as I knew it before would never be the same. My dad's death set in motion a profound awakening for me. I needed to be stronger for a bigger purpose. Mark needed me. Ann needed me. I needed myself.

SECTION 2 - DOCTORS & MEMORY LOSS

SECTION 2 - DOCTORS & MEMORY LOSS

Chapter 14: Realization
[2010]

Since my brother, Allen, was out of the country, I had the primary responsibility for cleaning out Dad's apartment, deciding on three piles, one to be kept for the family, artwork to be donated, and clothing to be distributed to thrift stores. My father had several oil paintings he painted over the years and never sold, landscapes, religious scenes, with Jesus, Mary and Joseph surrounded by angels, also large animals, such as horses and tigers, and varieties of birds and eagles. If anyone thinks it is possible to go through your beloved parents' treasures, to sort and place value on artwork expressed with meticulous care from a father you adored, it's not.

I found the task gut-wrenching and simply at the end of each lonely-as-sin day, unbearable. I wiped my eyes to stone with the back of my arm in his apartment, cleaned out tissue boxes as salty tears ran beneath my eyes, sat on his bed with rubber limbs and cold feet. No matter what I told myself, I can do this, I can cope with this-it was me sitting with the hollowed-core emptiness of a mannequin, far from reason or hope or sanity.

Sitting on the bare tile floor in the kitchen, I stared out the dining room window. My hands were sore, the tiny muscles in my palms in spasm, sick of moving, sorting, holding, or pinching.

Inside his office room, he kept a tin file box with important papers he always reminded me about, in case anything happened. Inside were love letters to my mom. Reading them, finger stroking page after page for hours heart forced me to dig deep to continue. When does a body run out of tears?

After I finished the final dusting, sweeping, vacuuming, mopping (making me the Mrs. Clean of sterilization and scented cleaning products), I contacted the resident manager for a refund on the deposit for my father's clean apartment. To my shock, the manager said they had to keep part of it, as she replied, "The apartment had an odor." I told her it must be the garbage disposal.

"Nope," she said tartly. "It wasn't the garbage disposal."

SECTION 2 - DOCTORS & MEMORY LOSS

A sudden rush of rage made me tremble. The apartment was clean for days since my dad passed inside it. Incensed, I wrote a concise complaint letter to the general manager. They apologized by giving a full refund.

Previously, I felt I carried the role of support and caregiver for my mother and father since my brother, Allen, lived out of town after his marriage. He rarely visited our parents in Fresno because he worked hard, and was totally devoted to his new family. While my Mark was sick, and as the weeks progressed after I released the apartment to the manager, handing in dad's keys with a gasp, I became over-sensitive to my brother's absence. Frankly, even though happy for him and his new life, it left me a little out in the cold. My new life consumed my being.

Do I quit work to take care of Mark? I had major decisions to make. I didn't know if my retirement was enough to sustain me, if-when-if-when-if-when Mark passed. Since I was the sole caregiver for Mark, I wondered if I could apply for disability benefits instead of regular Social Security? Answer - Advised I would not qualify because I was his spouse, able-bodied, mentally competent, and not the one with a disability.

"But I need financial help, and stressed to my limits."

"I'm sorry," the disability rep commented. "You must have a physical injury to qualify."

"We've paid in for decades."

"Doesn't matter."

"Well, what financial program is available for the caregiver spouses? To help them out. Who would I call?"

"You're asking if there is financial assistance for you, the able-bodied spouse."

"Yes."

"To take care of their sick husband or wife? Like a skilled nurse?"

"Yes. Our second marriage, we don't share assets." A pause, and a further pause.

"Hello?" I said.

Through my diligent efforts - meaning I floundered through mounds of confusing research, like a fish flopping on land - I found out that an individual could qualify for Medi-Cal if they made under a certain amount in social security income. The government would pay for skilled nursing up to

SECTION 2 - DOCTORS & MEMORY LOSS

the median cost of $7,290 for a semi-private room, less their social security dollar amount, in a care facility. Recent numbers from senioradvisor.com, as of 9/18 for a semi-private room, states an average number of $243 daily or $7,290 monthly. It didn't make sense to me the government would rather pay to have the patient in a month skilled nursing facility than to subsidize the family, who is caregiving for the ill family member at home by an additional $2,000 per month.

The data numbers I gathered were staggering, with the population of baby boomers reaching the twilight age. Severe illnesses kept them home with caregivers, who, from the emotional and psychological stress or health problems, ended up dying before the severely ill spouse or family member. Sometimes, caregivers seemed to require more help, support, and financial resources than the loved ones.

I had wonderful family members, Mark's brother and his wife, Mark's sister and my daughter, Ann. His daughters, Jill and Tammy lived five hours away, one with three small children and one starting her family. Even though they expressed a willingness to help, it was unfathomable to think they could pitch in five hours away. They sent emails and called. I asked them to take turns and alternate their visits to their dad, even if it was every two months. Not many visits came, both busy in their lives and five hours away. They each managed to come and pitch in twice. He always asked, "Why don't the girls call me or come visit?"

"I know your girls love you, but they have busy lives."

I tried to keep peace with my faith, and continuing prayers to God, it kept me steady, but I got angry at times. His daughters invited us to visit them. They didn't understand how difficult it was to drive and more difficult to take Mark out of his routine. Even though we visited his daughters (loving with all of his heart), he was confused and troubled within different surroundings away from home.

Twice we took the train south to visit his daughters, though long and exhausting. Our travel route went like this: train for two hours, transfer to a bus in Bakersfield for one and a half hours, drive through the L. A. Grapevine, and wait in a busy terminal in Los Angeles for one hour to catch a second train, if lucky. Not only was the trip long, I worried when I went to the bathroom. I gave Mark instructions to stay seated, but couldn't relax, thinking he'd forget and wander off, get lost and disoriented. He shuffled off in a hardware store once before, so it made me uneasy. We only made that kind of balls to the wall trip twice.

Mark did not do well. He was ready to come home on the second day of those visits. How did Mark feel inside? Physically with us, at times distant, as though he listened to someone else in the room. What did these transparent people say or direct him to think and do?

My conversations with his daughters didn't go well.

"You can see how hard it is," I said at the kitchen table in Tammy's house.

"I'm sure it is tough," Tammy said, feigning understanding.

"It's more than that," I said. "It's impossible."

She nodded as if empathy alone would get her out of it. After a while, I stopped trying with them.

I remember when we returned home, train-bus-train, wondering why he was beyond aloof, day and night. If anyone was home inside his being, I couldn't find him. Led away by the disease, the internal terrorists made people do crazy things. I often thought, What is it that people or seniors do, who don't have help or support to monitor what they have or what they are doing? How is it that people with Dementia or Alzheimer's just walk into traffic? They are innocent. Most do not understand how, when someone is crushed by a car while walking across a speeding highway, how it could happen.

SECTION 2 - DOCTORS & MEMORY LOSS

Chapter 15: Wellness Clinic Exit
[2010]

In the interim of all things chaotic and dehumanizing, we left the alternative clinic mid-care because of my dad's death on June 10, 2010. I had to deal with the wellness clinic in some way; continue Mark's care, try like hell to save him from dying.

Until we heard different, Mark continued with supplements. It amazed me despite Mark's deteriorating condition; he trusted me, giving him the twenty-five pills, capsules, and tablets. He had a difficult time swallowing, choking on the pill after pill. Along with this program, was a prescription of a hormone cream, that I spread on his arms with rubber gloves. I teased him I might start growing a beard if it got on me.

"No beard for you," he said. "You're the most beautiful woman I've ever loved."

I tried to call the doctor at the clinic, but difficult to reach her by phone. I faxed her a letter and asked for assistance. She responded and requested our return to the clinic to finish. A pall of hideous fatigue washed over me. I didn't want to go back. Mark didn't want to go back. It was difficult, dog-paddling like crazy for any ounce of energy, to survive what became sheer exhaustion alone, and not survivable. I loathed to rehashing the long 10-hour days and the difficult task of making sure Mark could handle it all.

After much contemplation, I decided it was too much for us to handle. In my gut, this new regimen of supplements and treatments didn't help. I made a dreaded call to cancel the remainder of the treatments. I was afraid the internal terrorist already invaded too much of his brain. I was derelict. A sinner. A possible gold digger in his daughters' eyes. Negligent. Foolish. Dumb. A token wife without a clue.

And with the reality understood of my precious husband slipping away from me, a woman and wife, soon to be forever alone. There was nothing for it. No miracle. No sudden pot of gold to materialize at the last second like in the movies. We would not pass 'Go,' on the Memory

SECTION 2 - DOCTORS & MEMORY LOSS

Loss Monopoly board. My life's mission was simple at the end of all things sad and painful.

I made the remainder of his so-called useful life as meaningful as I could. He depended on me and trusted me with all his heart. They had not taken his heart. I experienced his true love, in the way he looked at me and accepted me, with all my faults. He was my joy, and I was his peace. We would do this together. It was an ugly business of living and dying in our house together, as a devoted husband and wife. However, we would continue to walk in the same sad circles in the same bad dream, until one of us stopped.

Caregivers often died from stress before the sick spouse.

A response from the assigned doctor told me she would send me medications to transition Mark from the detox he was on since she wouldn't help over the phone.

I answered the door a couple of days later to a Fed Ex carrier. When I opened the box, I couldn't believe what I saw. Doctor prescribed several boxes of syringes and meds to administer to Mark. Pushed away and sent off with a modicum of care, so it all appeared legal, above board and necessary should anyone mention malpractice. I was so sick and lonely, I wondered how my heart would stand the pressure. The medications came with vague instructions, unclear doses, and possible side effects. I wasn't a nurse, or a healer. Glaring at the box of syringes and needles, the unforeseen smell of alcohol invaded my nostrils. I was not considered anything by the state of California except for a second wife with assets that remained separate from her second husband's assets. I hated the smell: Door Guard and Needle Stabber, Warden and Haggard Doctor. New terms added to my list of hell.

As I transitioned Mark from the wellness clinic's treatments, I waited a few months before settling my dad's estate.

I didn't know whether to blame the alternative clinic's doctor or the pharmacy. I fired a fax to the female doctor about the lack of instruction; and that I was not paying for the syringes. I called the pharmacy to complain about the inadequate or non-existent direction. It was too overwhelming to handle. If this was a psych ward set in a movie, this was the line in the script stating; a woman loses it.

While I worked on the allocation of financial distributions between my brother and me, the gardener came to the front door. He told me he inadvertently left the gate open, and our puppy, Barni, a feisty King Charles Cavalier, got out. Fortunately, one of his men retrieved him. My chest pounded like I had a heart attack from the stress of everything. I didn't know which direction to go from time to time. I yelled at the gardener in the best Spanish I knew, which was slowly telling them in English, "You better be more careful next time, or you won't have a job!"

After they left, I felt terrible for yelling at them. Mark sat in a chair without any motion, his back to me, facing our garden outside. He didn't realize there was a problem and that the puppy was gone.

The doorbell rang. I went to the door, completely forgetting I called a sprinkler guy for the leaky faucet in the yard. I answered the door with Barni in my arms. He loved our puppy and petted him. He said he and his wife had a beagle dog that needed a brother or sister. After he left, a light went on. As much as I loved Barni and was my elixir at times, I needed to find him a home. I couldn't give him the attention he needed with everything else. After yelling at the gardener, the doctor, and the pharmacy, I had to lighten my load. It broke my heart, losing my dad broke my heart, and losing Mark was breaking my heart.

"Hi," I said. "This is Jean. You just helped me with my sprinkler? Would you and your wife be interested in my King Charles Cavalier puppy? I'm having a hard time with everything. I can't risk him getting out or give him the attention he deserves."

The sprinkler guy came over with his wife. Barni jumped all over them, kissed, and licked them, almost saying, "Take me." They asked me to take Barni to meet their dog. At their house was the first time I saw Barni cower in front of anyone, their dog was the Alpha. They soon became fast friends. Barni had a new home.

Everything Barni was to me, was encouragement and love. He followed me everywhere, diligently, and showered me with kisses and licks. He helped me through my sorrow of losing my dad, and finally, I grieved for both my dad and my precious puppy. I went home and sobbed for days to purge all my losses. It didn't work. Mostly after weeks of crying, I only felt numb and missed my sweet loving King Charles Cavalier puppy.

To cope, I reached out to people I had not contacted for years. My out of town high school friend, Sara, was full of personality, smiles, and comfort. She made trips to see her family and often stopped to visit. She saw my significant responsibility and offered to help out. If I took Mark on a trip, Sara offered to go with us. It was a great offer, and I seriously considered it. Having a supportive friend who would travel with us would help tremendously.

Mark wanted to go on an Alaskan cruise, and I wanted to make it happen. I invited his brother, Robert, and his wife, Fran. Together, we went to the travel agent and looked at different brochures. It was much to take in. I wasn't sure about it. They wanted to go but suddenly canceled. I feared they thought Mark was too far gone. I wanted to try the trip anyway. After a few weeks, my intuition nagged me, maybe not a good idea. I didn't know how to break it to Mark until one evening. While watching repeats of last years' weather channel in bed, my help came. The show focused on inclement weather, with fishermen on their boat out at sea in Alaska sliding from side to side and water splashing everywhere.

"Jean, I don't think we should go, the weather looks pretty bad," Mark said.

"I agree, we'll do something else." I couldn't believe it. His short-term memory loss, but he remembered the pending trip. I thought this is a saving grace from God. God is saving me.

I later planned a trip to our Maui timeshare, our last weeklong vacation, difficult because it required airplane transportation. I invited Sara to come along. Mark enjoyed a fun social life but became insecure. At the beach or dinner, Sara stayed with him while I left to use the bathroom. He was nervous each time, turning his head to look for me. After that vacation, it was short trips within proximity to home. Maui was our last significant flight and travel adventure together.

* * *

SECTION 2 - DOCTORS & MEMORY LOSS

During this time, my high school friend Janie struggled with an illness that mimicked Parkinson's disease. At 60, her prognosis was sketchy, diagnosed with a rare disease, Nuclear Palsy, and admitted to an assisted living facility in Palm Desert, California.

Janie introduced me to my first husband. I reminisced about Janie, my great Irish friend, a petite, blue-eyed, artistic, blond darling with humor so quick she made the Irish laugh from their graves. We went to a private Catholic school together. She was creative and had a special affinity toward my father, a sisterhood to my artistic father.

I had to visit her, so I asked Mark's daughters to pitch in. The youngest daughter, Tammy, came from southern California and took her dad to the older daughters in northern California for the weekend. It took extra work to get his things together, pills for the next few days, and instructions. They brought him home early on Sunday. So, I made arrangements for his sister, Pauline, to cover until I arrived.

I asked Sara to visit our friend. Her cheerful face was the best company for this first trip away from Mark, and a much needed time away. We made the five-hour drive and drove directly to the assisted living home to see our buddy.

When we arrived, we walked down a hallway and saw old residents, some in walkers, wheelchairs, listless in bed, stoic, but some smiling toothless and seemingly happy, a memory embedded in my mind for a long time. The friendly staff directed us to our delicate, aging friend, with short gray hair and no teeth. Janie always prided herself with lush, thick hair, always coiffured perfectly. We were both taken aback with a lump of emotion, somewhere between our hearts and stomachs. Janie smiled at us and, after hugs, led us outside to visit. After reminiscing about old times, we asked her if she wanted something special for dinner.

Without hesitation, Janie yelled out, "Steak and lobster! The food is boring here."

We had our mission, shopped for new blouses for our dear friend, and searched for the desired steak and lobster meal. We called several restaurants, but the lobster was not in season, so we ordered steak and king crab. The temperature reached 115 to 120 degrees during the summer.

SECTION 2 - DOCTORS & MEMORY LOSS

When we returned, we took turns feeding her. Somehow Sara, a vegetarian, was positioned next to the steak to cut the steak and fed Janie. I cracked the crab, pulled it from its shell, dipped it in butter, and fed it to Janie Moroccan-style, as butter dripped from her chin. It was her last meal, and we couldn't get it to her fast enough. After dinner, we left, and the hugs began. Janie hugged me and whispered, "See you in Heaven."

I held back tears, at the same time, knew one day we'd end up together. As difficult as it was, we gave our dear friend the best goodbye possible. I was glad Sara offered to drive. I relaxed in the car before getting home. I sifted through memories of good times and wished we could have spent more time with Janie. However, knowing how difficult it was for Mark with me gone, in some way, made me eager to get home.

Pauline greeted me with a hug, and I began to get reports of how the weekend went with Mark's daughters and their dad. He had a great visit with his daughters and his grandchildren. I didn't know any details; however, I'm sure it got confusing with the repeated conversations. I heard how difficult it was to give him his pills because he only swallowed one pill at a time. I knew what they experienced, and in some ways, I was glad they did. At least they saw our daily new normal.

I received a call from his concerned younger daughter, Tammy. Out of nowhere, her father went into the garage and looked at a pair of long, sharp pruning shears. She detoured him away from the garage until I arrived. I had to keep him out of the garage until I hid all the questionable, dangerous tools.

* * *

Two months later, the first respite invitation came from my friend Sara to visit in Reno, Nevada. I hated driving in the mountains, a fear I never understood. I had never driven to Reno, but I thought I needed to challenge myself out of my cozy comfort zone and make that drive. Plus, I feared I was going nuts beneath the continual grind and workload.

I had to organize a plan for three full days for the family with Mark. I commissioned my brother-in-law, Robert, sister-in-law, Pauline, and Ann to be with him. I hand-wrote an itinerary with phone numbers for Mark, so

SECTION 2 - DOCTORS & MEMORY LOSS

he could see where I was throughout the weekend. I kept doing an internal exercise to psyche myself about the drive. Sara said she would give me a grand tour of Reno and the old town of Carson City, with all the history, saloons and ghosts. It didn't matter where we went, I just needed a change of pace, girl talk and hopefully slept through the night.

I left the house anxious and jittery but left Mark. Robert came to be with Mark Friday. I felt the same emptiness in my heart that I felt the first time I left Ann as a toddler with my mom, as a parent. But now, instead of dropping off my child for the weekend, it was my spouse. The shift from sunny days of love and passion to peek-a-boo days of gray, foggy love and responsibility revealed itself. I wasn't always sure if I gauged my senses, for the pure shock and shifted each day of the random acts of potential danger I observed from Mark. I loved my husband, but in a different capacity, as a caregiver for a child-like partner. I went into the car and sat with a bucket-load of hesitation. I heard the phone inside and ran back in.

"Hi! You on your way?" Sara asked.

"Ready or not, yes, I'm leaving," I said.

"Enjoy the scenery."

I didn't understand what she meant until I got on the road. I approached the mountains with ongoing construction, and a fork in the street, one low and one high. The low way had many semi-trucks with loads, which I preferred. I knew it would delay my time, so I decided on the high road. BIG MISTAKE! The high road ended up on a very skinny, narrow lane, between highway walls on both sides. I crept along, and my hand gripped the steering wheel so tight, as though I was walking on a thin tight rope, trying to balance and not fall. A car behind me honked. My heart almost pounded to the steering wheel, I decided to calm myself with deep inhalations and exhalations while praying, Dear God, please get me there safely. It was a long road, but I finally arrived and had my respite weekend, and felt a sort of independence for that challenging drive. Whew! I had time alone to think, breath, and re-boot.

Ann planned to pick up Mark on Saturday afternoon and took him to her house for dinner. She planned a birthday dinner for her dad and wanted to include Mark in the dinner party. She later told me Mark carried the itinerary the entire time and kept looking at it. It was a very tough weekend for him without me. The future had to include him on short getaways, as long as he could.

Robert told me later when he saw my car gone from the garage and said, "Her car's gone, she left me."

* * *

An invitation came from Sara to stay at a mutual friend's home in Carmel. It was a beautiful home on the ocean with two-tier steps up to the house. After we arrived, I made sure Mark was upstairs and safe. I began unloading our luggage. After going up and down three times, I remember thinking that it wasn't supposed to be this way, he's my warrior, taken over by the internal terrorist. I'm the warrior, and I can't stand it.

After we got settled in, I found Mark going through the bedroom drawers of our friend's home. I watched him the entire time. I worried he might try to walk down the stairs without me and go for a walk. Sara was a good friend and kept watch while I showered or was unavailable in the bathroom. While there, another girlfriend, Mary, invited us to dinner. I didn't want to drive at night. So, her husband offered to take us to their home. Asked to go outside for drinks and appetizers, we sat on their deck with a view of the Pacific Ocean, eating appetizers of warm garlic toast, capers, and smoked salmon. The ocean chill brushed our face, while we looked at their garden landscape with native, exotic plants with round orange flowers, called pin cushions swaying with the breeze.

Mark rarely took off his jacket, even when we sat for dinner. He was still sociable, but his facial expressions changed since being on his medication, looked stressed and uncomfortable, rarely smiling. Eating bites of butter and spoons of horseradish, everything slower, and usually the last one to finish. When he inadvertently took their cloth napkin and put it in his pocket. I made a mental note: I'll have to wash it and mail it back to Mary. I never mentioned it to him. Dignity was everything.

* * *

SECTION 2 - DOCTORS & MEMORY LOSS

A few months later, at home, I planned a weekend away with Mark for a change of scenery. I sat at the computer in the home office and searched for our timeshare availability. Mark walked in periodically and asked, "What ya doing?"

"How about a weekend in Napa Valley? We could do a spa day and have a couples massage." I said.

"That would be nice," he answered but looked at me confused.

I found a nice weekend getaway at a Sonoma spa. I thought it would do us some good. On the morning of our spa appointment, I woke to let Mark know we needed to get ready for our massage at 9:00. He looked aloof and said he didn't want to go. We did have a lovely corner cottage with a fireplace and windows with a view of fragrant roses from all sides. I tried to sweeten the activity and said, "There's a fireplace in the spa, and we can have breakfast and coffee near their fireplace, afterward. It'll be fun."

He finally agreed. I later discovered why. I walked him to the men's locker room and said, "Change your clothes and put one of their robes on."

I proceeded to the ladies' room to put my robe on. After waiting several minutes, I talked to the attendant about his illness. I asked the attendant to go in and make sure there were no other men in the dressing room so that I could assist him.

"It's ok for you to go in," she said.

I walked in to see him. When I entered, he stood there in the locker room, almost in tears. I wanted to cry after I saw him. Mark couldn't remember what to do. I tried to reassure him and helped him undress to put the robe on.

"I'm going to the massage room with you. It'll be a nice relaxing time, and then we can sit in the waiting room and have coffee and Danish pastry near the fireplace. I'll be with you the whole time. You won't be alone." I said.

"Ok," He said.

He looked broken and sad, with his eyes and lips dropped down to the ground. It killed my heart to see him so vulnerable. I thought he would enjoy it, and instead, it tortured him.

The internal terrorist had him. It directed his brain to stop exercising, stop gardening, and to stop having a desire to fish and travel. The only thing it didn't take was his heart. It didn't matter who we were with; Mark praised me for being a great driver, smart person, and a great wife. He wanted me with him all the time. In the beginning, while he still had his driver's license, the doctor suggested I start going to the driver's side of our SUV.

One time we went to some friends for dinner. I got in the driver's seat.

"What are you doing?" He followed me, thinking he would drive, then frowned.

"Please let me drive. I never get to drive." I said, and he succumbed.

"Ok," he replied while he walked to the passenger side. Dignity. Dignity.

"I need to learn to drive better at night. You can help me." I said.

SECTION 2 - DOCTORS & MEMORY LOSS

Chapter 16: Hallucinations
[2011]

At home, I used to see our wicker trays as decorative and obscure, used only for guests. But they became part of our new ritual of togetherness. They held the confidence of our new normal, while we broke bread for lunch and dinner. They also served in giving Mark all his new many meds. He slowly choked down one pill at a time, as if tasting the despised Brussel sprouts of his childhood meal. I couldn't blame him.

During this winter of 2011, after he got sick, I visualized the winters when a crackling fire burned, while we enjoyed our glass of wine, cheese, and fruit before our dinner.

Walking in and out of the room to check on my husband became sequential. Mark was always helpful in the house. When it was time for dinner, he asked, "How many are staying for dinner?" I thought, does he think my dad is coming over? I wanted to pretend his escalating hallucinations did not exist, but the internal terrorist directed him.

I had no say. Powerless. To stop it, alter it, run after it, withdraw from it. Powerless.

The kitchen used to permeate the house sometimes with the aroma of a roast or homemade chicken soup with garlic, carrots, celery, and potatoes. Instead, it became the fast-food counter, which served sporadically from white takeout boxes. I couldn't spend time away from him because I fear he'd walk out the door and get lost.

I called him and got no reply, so I quickly wiped my apron to get the onion from our sandwiches off my fingers. As I walked back into the living room, he was gone. I panicked and ran through the hallway to the bedroom. He stood in front of his closet.

"What are you doing in the closet? I asked.

"I'm looking for a shirt for the guy in the living room. He says he needs a shirt," he said.

"Who?" I asked.

"The man. On our couch."

SECTION 2 - DOCTORS & MEMORY LOSS

There was no one else in our house. My husband looked tense, emotionless, and almost preoccupied. Even though I cleaned out his closet to simplify things, I imagined this was still confusing for him, he opened the sliding doors to the closet, looking at the numerous button-down plaid shirts, deciding which one to part with, and would fit this stranger in the living room. I couldn't believe what he told me. I wondered if I was having a nightmare. I opened my eyes, then closed them, held them closed, and then opened them. I believed if he did recognize this unknown person, then maybe he didn't want to alarm me. I tried to stay calm and held back tears, raised my eyebrows, and pressed my lips, while this lost soul sat in our house. I went with it, all of it. I had to.

"That's nice, but let's not do this right now. I'll help you later after we have our dinner."

As I walked him back into the living room, I thought, maybe I should have asked him about this guy. But I couldn't bring myself to do it. Does he believe I see this guy? Is this guy a lost spirit from the other side of our physical world? He sounds like a harmless soul, but I'm terrified. The stranger was in our private space. Where did he come from? Who was he? What did he look like? You see, it was months I'd adapted to Mark's vision of his world, hoping to understand it, interfacing where I was wanted, and staying outside of it when I was pushed away by Mark. From my love for Mark, I attempted to become one with him and one with his internal terrorist, so that I would be included. See what he saw. Feel what he felt. Morph into a wife who would travel with Mark into all of his hidden worlds and universes. I failed miserably.

Mark became stone-faced, preoccupied, and aloof. I monitored all his actions in the house, unable to leave him alone anymore.
He used to love to shower in our newly remodeled bathroom with the large tiles under the new rainfall nozzle, but he didn't like showers anymore. He wouldn't go in alone. Being an adventurer and hunter in exotic places, he never feared anything. He was terrified and called me in and said, "They are laughing at me."

I offered to stay in the bathroom with him while he showered. He told me he closed his eyes, thinking they would go away, but instead, they

SECTION 2 - DOCTORS & MEMORY LOSS

laughed and pointed at him, to the point of scaring him in an urgent need to relieve himself.

My mind burned to be inside his head and I imagined how the strangers might look. It was all imagination, but in my exhausted state, imagination was a friend I often ran to with open arms.

If this were a science fiction movie, I was the highly regarded psychiatrist telepath.

"Is it a go? Am I ready?"

Imagine ten scientists, doctors, engineers and security guards behind the glass-walled computer room that had my back should anything go wrong. And I trusted them implicitly. My job was of the highest security clearance; meant for those associated with loved ones who have been infiltrated by an invasion of an internal terrorist.

A shower of mist surrounded me. I'd learn Mark's thoughts through water, through the conduction of his memories. The water shower contained the same wave frequency as the water inside his brain cells.

"Ready," I concluded settling into my chair. Water sounds magnified.

If it became too painful the team would allow me to back out.

"I can handle it."

"I mean it, Jean. No playing hero. You could be damaged."

"I know the risks. Don't lecture me.

Counting down to mind entry...five-four-three-two-one...

My imagination starts going wild with beings, who might look like alien characters with translucent colors, an aura around their whole body, a thickness of six inches wide.

My eyes shut; my mind starts to see...

A thin iridescent light shining outside of their entire body, outlining their head, shoulders, arms, naked, pale, broad, hairless and shiny chest, torso, legs, feet, front, back, and even their lipless, earless face. The light looks like an untouchable, protective veil that would burn you to black if you tried touching them. Their bodies with eyes golden, round and flickering lights, absorbing colors in the room. One might have a commanding demeanor, with a fiery reddish, flickering light all around his body, no hair, bending his head to get through the doorway. With a deep, heavy and wicked laughter, like he could consume the entire space with

SECTION 2 - DOCTORS & MEMORY LOSS

fire. Another man with an amber light around his bottom half and a clear light on top, meeker, shorter, with a higher pitched voice, alternating his laughter in between the dominant reddish man. Maybe a soft pink small presence with long, golden, string-like, mop-like, strands hanging from the top of what looks like a petite, slender woman, with a soft, but continuous laughter, like a hyena. All of them, moving by electrical, radioactive mechanical materials, with robotic-like voices, sounding as if it's coming out of a chamber, with loud vibrational tones.

"Jean! Jean wake up! Brain waves are spiking. You have to wake up!"

"…loud tones. Do you have it? I'm coming out now."

"Hurry, Jean." Mark yells.

"Prepare for separation. Mark, I love you."

"…wake her up damnit. Spiking!"

"Understood. Disconnect water spray. Separation in five-four-three-two-one…"

I wake up to applause from the computer room. I wake up to cheers that I am the strongest woman psychiatrist telepathic bitch in the world.

Hesitantly, as if he might be eaten, Mark steps out of the shower.

We went on. My husband was unable to pay attention to anything for very long. I went along when he told me about the invisible people. I didn't understand why they were here. I couldn't bring myself to ask him what they looked like and if they looked like us. They haunted us. They were frightening and unpredictable people acting more like vampire creatures, who showed up and were ready to strike at any time.

An article from NPR review said hallucinations are not uncommon; up to 50 percent of people with Alzheimer's disease experienced hallucinations, delusions or psychotic symptoms. One suffering from Early Onset Alzheimer's shared his experience of seeing spider-like forms floating in peripheral vision, lions and birds, sprays of blood among the spiders and a bird flying in tighter and tighter circles, then all of a sudden, beak first, darts in almost suicide mission explosions inside his heart. Another Alzheimer's article stated an Alzheimer's patient saw flashing lights, with complex, strange situations of brightly colored people or animals.

I wasn't a psychiatrist or a telepath or special or smart or savvy or strong.

SECTION 2 - DOCTORS & MEMORY LOSS

I was just Jean. The woman who loved Mark.
It wasn't enough. I wasn't enough.

SECTION 2 - DOCTORS & MEMORY LOSS

SECTION 2 - DOCTORS & MEMORY LOSS

Chapter 17: Family Notifications
[2011]

A few months before Mark's birthday in November 2011, he became incontinent and embarrassed, a humiliated face about his wet pants, as though it was his fault. He took deep breaths as his shoulders raised up and down.

"Mark, it's okay, it's not your fault. Let's change your pants." I tapped his shoulders and hugged him.

Another phase, I thought, but how would I suggest he wear new disposable underwear.? What kind would I buy? There were two choices at the drug store, plain white diaper-looking "Huggies," and the adult kind, gray color with a slight pattern, which I eventually chose. I bought the underwear and went home, then laid them on the bed. I tried to make it fun, so I said to him, "Mark, what do you think of this sexy underwear? Can you try them on?" He smiled, and he was game.

"If it's okay with you, I'm throwing the old underwear away. That way, you can start wearing new underwear. They will work better." He nodded by robotically moving his head up and down.

We loved the setting of our family room, and our furniture after our remodel a few years ago. It faced our deck and backyard. One day, we sat on the living room sofa. Mark looked at me and said, "This house is nice, but when are we going home?" I didn't know how to answer him. But it was a signal. It couldn't have been clearer if God had struck me with a bolt of lightning. We were at home. And we were never going home together again.

As days went by, his back hurt more and more. He walked with a gait in his leg. He woke and wanted to leave his pajamas on all day, a long T-shirt and print cotton pants. He didn't want to shower, so I left him alone. I found him later in the day, standing in front of the closet, looking at his shirts. I asked, "Do you want to shower and dress now?"

"No."

"We need to change your underwear at least."

"No, I don't want to change."

SECTION 2 - DOCTORS & MEMORY LOSS

About a half-hour later in the living room, I smelled his underwear. I said, "Mark, why don't we take a shower together? I can wash your hair and massage your scalp." He finally agreed, but still very confused that day. Things were speeding up; his deterioration progressed too fast. I wasn't sure if we would be able to continue in the same way with our life. I needed help. I was afraid he would be combative again. If he hit or struck me in the temple, I might blackout. I couldn't risk it.

* * *

Since his birthday was right after Christmas, I wanted it to be a special birthday and have a small open house. I invited some of his friends and hosted another dinner celebration with his kids. I wanted Mark to have quality time with each of them.

His friends came and spent time with their dear friend. A wine bar and tables set outside near tall large heater lamps kept people warm. Our chef friend, Shelley, made gourmet flatbread pizzas, and many appetizers of cheese, meats, fruits, and salads, all presented beautifully. Mark didn't want to change and wore his uniform, worn about every day: his baseball hat, fleece jacket, and jeans. The marks and effects of the medication, his sullen expression, and stoned eyes on his face. In spite of it, everyone gave him love and attention. An open house, but everyone stayed for hours, standing room only with friends and family sitting on every place available inside and out on the patio.

His two daughters, with their families, visited for his birthday dinner at Mark's favorite Italian restaurant days after Christmas. When it was time to order, I asked Mark what he wanted for dinner. Even though we had been to the restaurant many times, Mark asked me to order for him. His daughters looked with knowing and sad eyes and saw the change in their father's eyes, bewildered, trapped, alone, blank. He still smiled and had small exchanges with his grandchildren, but it was evident he didn't have his spark and energy.

During their visit, I had an opportunity to have a brief conversation with Mark's son-in-law, John. He listened with full attention, as I confided things progressed faster than we thought, and it was becoming difficult to manage. It was time to have written communication with his daughters. My note said:

"I had a brief conversation with John while you were here for your dad's birthday. I'm sure you realize after seeing your dad, his illness has progressed faster than we thought. His personality has always been loving, kind, and sweet, but it changes randomly. I don't blame him, his physical health is not good, every day something aches, or he has trouble with his asthma. He has gone through testing of just about everything ailing him, and it's very exhausting. As you can imagine, as frustrating as it is for him, it is frustrating for me. Advised by the doctor to lock up all meds and anything harmful months ago, I finally did. He has hoarded things in the house in odd places, including food, nasal sprays, even backup supplies that I had in my closet, Christmas decorations, several pairs of sunglasses, etc.

He hallucinates at times and made comments about people in our house.

Then, he looked in his closet and told me he was looking for a shirt for the man on the sofa who said he needed a shirt. It scared me, but I went along with him.

I contacted our neurologist and a doctor at the Alzheimer's Center to ask for advice and help. Your dad just had his appointment with his neurologist for another test. He went down from last July 2011, at number 22 (out of 30) to 16. I told his neurologist he was acting depressed. She suggested I let the family know, and ask them to check-in with him to reassure him, even if only for 5 minutes. He gets insecure when he doesn't have communication from you; he loves you so much. I know logistically it is difficult for you, but if you could call and check-in, and cards would also help.

Consequently, I have been taking your dad to daycare at an Assisted Living Facility for Alzheimer's, on a day-by-day basis, starting with half days and a couple of whole days. He has enjoyed it most of the time. I thought the social interaction and program offered could give him a change of pace, and give me some relief. I'm introducing him slowly to all this. He is so used to going everywhere with me on errands, but lately, he has been reluctant to do so. The doctor at the Alzheimer's Center said the activities program would be good for him. After he gets there, he seems to enjoy it. I've been talking to the activities people, and they say he is enjoying the social aspect of it, but not so much the games. I've been telling him they enjoy his stories and sense of humor. I also tell him it helps me when he can go, so I don't have to drag him along.

His illness has been challenging and sad for me. I didn't think this would happen so fast. I know what is inevitable in the future, but I'm trying to ease both of us into this transition in baby steps.

It's a sick, strange disease. Your dad still remembers my dad died, and where he last lived. Every time we pass the intersection where we turned to his place, your dad takes his hat off and salutes him. Mentioning that, the other day, he asked me if we were moving back home. The doctor said off-days will occur, and then, seem all right the next day. Nothing in the classes can prepare anyone for this, as it is heartbreaking.

I'm doing the best I can in a situation we didn't choose. You can call my cell phone anytime or email me. Love, Jean."

* * *

I called my brother-in-law, Robert, and sister-in-law, Pauline, to update them on the need for Mark's transition. His brother agreed it was time to start looking at options for assisted living facilities. Previously we all looked at places for Mark's mother, but this would be different and emotional. It was mind-shattering to think of my fit, good-looking, quick-witted Mark, spending time with the geriatric group. How would I explain it to him? I decided the whole experience had to be in baby steps. I was glad I found an assisted living place for Alzheimer's patients, five minutes away from our home. The facility had daycare activities, which were perfect for Mark. This also gave me a break away. Prior to all this, I took Mark everywhere with me. He even went to the hairdresser with me and sat for two hours waiting. On a Tuesday, I decided to tell him we were going shopping, then I said, "I met these people who need your help. It's a group of people who need to hear funny stories. It will help me if you could help them while I go on errands, then I'll be back to pick you up."

SECTION 2 - DOCTORS & MEMORY LOSS

I took him for 4 hours the first time. When I picked him up, I asked him if he had a nice time visiting, and Mark said, "Yes, I did."

The program started with-two afternoons per week for Mark. He didn't always want to go. At times, he needed help from the staff, to come out to the car and escort him inside the daycare facility. I always felt guilty at drop-off time. Looking back over the past six years, since he started showing signs of memory problems, this was only the third time I had a few hours to myself. I shouldn't have felt guilty, but I did. He was my husband, looked like my husband, but he'd become a dependent child.

SECTION 2 - DOCTORS & MEMORY LOSS

SECTION 2 - DOCTORS & MEMORY LOSS

Chapter 18: Movie Transition
[APRIL 2012]

Four months after Christmas in April 2012, on a Thursday, Mark continued to complain of his back hurting, so I asked him if it hurt when he urinated. He said, "A little."

I took him to his primary doctor for an evaluation. I thought he might have a possible urinary tract infection. Mark couldn't urinate for the lab analysis, so as a precaution, the doctor prescribed an antibiotic. I gave him the pills as prescribed.

The next day on Friday, I received a call from the occupational therapist. Mark's new walker arrived. Friday was usually the day I took Mark to a movie and an early dinner. Even though he was, in part, gone from me, I refused to let our romance or romantic gestures dwindle. Afterward, we went to test the walker at the doctor's office. With the help of the therapist, Mark seemed able to handle the new walker, so I asked him if he wanted to take his new walker to the movies, and he said, "Yes." My great outdoor man was blessed to have competent medical help, with doctors, occupational therapists and access to equipment like walkers. Yet, there I sat, viewing him from an internal distance as he maneuvered his walker in the medical office. He stooped, strained to push it, picked it up now and then to realign his course with a clunk or scrape or grunt on his part. It grew too hard for me to watch and I looked toward the floor, counting-counting-counting blessings so I wouldn't tear up.

I tried to keep things regular and kept up with our routine. None of our friends wanted to be shut-out and I kept them involved in our lives. On previous short trips to the Central California coast with good friends, I think Mark enjoyed being out, even though I oversaw him carefully, I 'think' because I don't know. I was never sure what was going on inside him. No matter my telepath skills, it was tough to keep playing 'guessing games' about his condition or mental clarity, and soon, I had to give it up. Caring the burden of 'pretend' for the sake of our friends, also became too much. I began to be honest instead of deflecting or rose-glassing things up.

SECTION 2 - DOCTORS & MEMORY LOSS

When asked how he was doing, I answered with a weary smile, I simply don't know.

During the day, while having lunch at a beach restaurant, I made sure that my friends kept watching outside the men's room. I feared he would wander off in an unfamiliar area. At a restaurant for dinner, he ate butter with his fork, and I had to cut his meat. Trying to be funny, I said, "You know butter is one of the major five food groups." I didn't care what anyone thought. I kept it mostly to the close friends who loved us and understood.

* * *

I took Mark to the movies every Friday. Since he loved animals, adventure, and nature, I selected the Disney movie, Chimpanzee. We pulled into the parking lot at Vista Cinemas in Fresno and finally found a spot. I watched him get out of the car, and then I handed him the new shiny aluminum, wide and sturdy walker. He didn't walk with it as he was instructed at the doctor's office, gliding instead of lifting or pushing, but instead, bent over like a deformed closet hanger, he took in a breath and heaved it like a grocery cart full of bags. He looked so winded and wobbly; I worried he might fall.

I heard 911 screamed inside my head. I didn't say it out. 911-911-911. HE CAN'T GET UP! My warped thoughts twisted around serious and comical commercials on television, where the person on the ground can't get up. In the background of my overly active imagination, the sound of howler monkeys in a jungle struck up a far distant cacophony swirled my war-trodden brain along with my dread and concern for Mark.

Operator for 911, what is your emergency?

My husband fell in the parking lot.

Where are you, Ma'am?

At the movies. Vista Cinemas Fresno.

Are you sure you're at the cinema and not the zoo? I can hear monkeys.

Monkeys? There are no monkeys?

Really! I can clearly hear them.

No, you can't. Oh, Lord. It is a dream! We're going to see CHIMPANZEE!!

SECTION 2 - DOCTORS & MEMORY LOSS

As I shook my head into submission, I said, gritting my teeth, "Maybe we should leave the walker this time. Let me help you, or maybe we should go home."

"No!" He yelled and struggled as if I were about to hit him, and he tried to move away.

By the time we made it to the lobby of the theatre, buffeted by a crowd of people, and managed the separate movie area, Mark fell. His knees went down to the ground as he tried to grip the handles, then his whole body stretched out. I dropped to the floor to help him when he yelled, "You pushed me! You pushed me. Why did you push me?" He said it too loud for my comfort.

My face felt zapped by a Taser. I tried to hold back tears, unable to lift him. Two men helped him up. I was mortified, embarrassed, and wondered if they thought I had pushed him. I leaned closer and whispered in his ear, "Mark, do you feel okay or should we leave?"

"I want to stay." He looked at me with no smile or emotion. His stare went right through me and gave me a chill. I kept hearing these words from the doctor: Don't challenge him; he might get combative. I was afraid but pissed. With his outburst and accusation, I couldn't take the chance of people thinking I abused him. I wanted to crawl into a hole and disappear.

In later weeks, I reflected on that incident and how hard I'd worked to keep things reasonable between us with routines, eating times, bedtimes, chores, errands, movies. Everything I read said to keep the interactive, social and ordinary things going. I watched him during the film off and on until he started to fall asleep.

I tried to escape in my thoughts during the movie. I thought about our mountain hiking trip to Tuolumne Meadows, right before our wedding in 2000, because I was desperate to recall anything at all to the 'goodness' around the man I married. I loved Mark.

We loved each other. But love wasn't working out for me anymore.

* * *

SECTION 2 - DOCTORS & MEMORY LOSS

September of 2000, before Mark and I married, he extended an invitation to go hiking in Tuolumne Meadows, near Yosemite Valley. I called it my boot camp. I believed Mark tested me. Previously, I handled our first few day hikes. This trip involved me organically in the raw, authentic self, no makeup involved, overnight with the outdoorsy group.

To the sporting goods store, we bought the right hiking boots, lightweight pants that zipped off at the knee when it was warm, and then re-zipped long for the cold, a heavier jacket, and a backpack.

Mark said it would be an excellent way of camping with permanent campsites, working bathrooms, showers, a wood-burning heater in each tent and a restaurant. He said, "Let's see what you're made of." One of his favorite sayings that became one of my favorite one-liners. I know he thought I was too prissy to do the outdoor stuff. Prissy, my ass, I thought. I'll show him.

I was determined to keep up, even though he was probably more physically fit than I was. I couldn't take any scent to attract bears: No makeup, perfume, deodorant, or lotion. We arrived at the meadows and got acclimated to the area. In the parking lot, campers and vehicles parked alongside large metal bins, which locked at night for any questionable items that couldn't be kept in our tents. Instructions not to keep anything with fragrance or food, not even gum or lotion could be kept in the cars, to prevent bear break-ins. In this area of wilderness, bears can literally, with their huge forearms and clawed feet, peel your car door off like peeling a banana, and they'll do it to get inside if they sniff food.

This high mountain adventure was heady. We hiked up hills in the wilderness, and I hoped to see a bear.

A centrally located wooden building with several windows adjacent to a creek and the cabins was the restaurant and reception area for all the hikers. We made reservations for dinner and our packed lunch for the next day hike. I had no idea what was in store for the next few days of hiking, but I was about to find out. We walked up a path to find our tent. Mark already told me, "This is the best way to camp. The tents are first class, with all the accommodations you have at home."

"Great," I said while I looked to see if he laughed, but he didn't.

SECTION 2 - DOCTORS & MEMORY LOSS

But I wondered why he made our tent sound like the Ritz Carlton. It turned out it was a permanent foundation, closed in with a canvas tent cover, a wood-burning heater, four twin beds with linens, blankets, a table with a candle, matches, and wood underneath. And yes, equipped with bathrooms and showers, fortunately not far away.

We got settled in our "exquisite" tent and started to explore the camp area. We took a short 5-mile hike on level ground from the camp and worked our way back as it approached dinner hour.

We saw families in the meadow with children, and we talked of bringing our respective adult children back to camp and hike this beautiful land. As we approached the restaurant, we walked near the creek, listened to the rush of water, and felt refreshed by the cool breeze. Everything that day at that very moment was so clear, pure, and mesmerizing. How lucky we both felt to be sharing this time at that place together.

Dusk approaching, we made our way back to the restaurant. Our table seated couples from different parts of the world. We heard many languages as people talked and laughed. Most spoke of the next day's hike up the mountain, with a higher elevation to the camp, cascading waterfalls, and the next night at a different site.

I hiked before but never envisioned a daunting hike like this one. We reached the campsite, and I was so relieved, but not for long. Mark always joked with me, and he confessed, "Jean, on this leg of the trip, we are in a tent with four beds, and we might have company, that is, if the campsite needs the extra space." I laughed and thought he was kidding. To my surprise, it wasn't long before we met our roommates, two gentlemen from San Francisco. In the fraternity of three men, I dealt with sleeping in the same tent with strangers. They slept on one side, head to feet, and then the other side with Mark and me across from them.

As we worked our way back and saw all the beautiful waterfalls, trees, landscapes, and blue skies, we talked of making this an annual trip with our extended families. We had time along the way to talk about our lives and our desires for the years ahead.

"I love you and don't want you to work so hard. Let's find you a job that would allow you more flexibility for our future travels. I saw an ad in the newspaper for a financial advisor. It's with a major national company." He said while we stopped for a break.

It was music to my ears. I leaned over to hug Mark.

* * *

"Let's go home," I whispered in the movie theatre after Mark fell asleep. He looked at me with a blank expression. After I touched his hand to hold it and help him up from his theater seat, he took my lead as I stood up, then he did.

"Okay," he responded. We quietly walked hand in hand, out a side exit door, with the walker folded under my arm, while I grasped Mark with my free hand and walked to the car into the parking lot.

We watched part of the movie about a curious three-year-old orphan chimpanzee, lost from his family, alone and hungry. Through nature's fate, a stranger, an older chimpanzee, found and adopted him, led, and showed him the way.

I attempted to find some sign from God in the movie; a positive message meant for me alone. Keep going! You can do it! Mark needs your help! I felt some connection and relief to God within the viewing of the movie. And I also heard monkeys grunting and squeaking, ramping up for jungle madness.

* * *

I quit work to care for Mark (No other option I would allow), I felt guilty for not serving home-cooked meals as often, but he couldn't be left alone long intervals unattended. After the Friday movie, I picked up dinner at a drive-through. He never complained about food, even before his illness.

After the ordeal at the theatre, we went to bed early that night, until I awakened. Usually, the time Mark woke to go to the bathroom, but he wasn't up. The new normal was waking up every three hours, often at midnight, 3:00 a.m., and 6:00 a.m. This night different, I woke at 3:00 with my body hot and sweaty. Mark was very still.

SECTION 2 - DOCTORS & MEMORY LOSS

"Are you awake?" I asked.

"Yes." He replied.

"I'm hot. Are you?" I asked.

"Yes," he said.

I touched his face and head, hot and clammy. I went to the bathroom and wet a washcloth for his forehead. Then, I grabbed a thermometer to take his temperature; it was 99. At that point, I asked, "Can I help take off your T-shirt to cool you?"

"I can't move." I tried to help, but he moaned with pain. I ran to the kitchen for scissors to cut his shirt off. Then I tried to lift his hips so I could take his wet underwear off, but he couldn't help. He said, "It hurts."

"Can you move anything?"

"I can't; it hurts."

"Where does it hurt?"

"My neck and my back."

"I'll cut your shirt off." I ripped the front of his underwear off and asked him if he could lift his butt to help me take his pants off.

"It hurts." He replied.

I called 911. The operator started questioning me. "Where does he hurt?"

"He's hot; he can't move his neck or his back. He can't even lift his hips."

The ambulance arrived, and the paramedics took his vitals right away. They asked for his symptoms. They explained they needed to keep his head straight with the sideboards and keep him straight on the stretcher. It was uncertain what caused his pain.

A helpless feeling, not knowing, and not being able to relieve him of his pain. I tried to stay calm. Up to this point, we went through at least six years of the progression of his disease, half of our marriage, relying on the professionals to guide us along this path, not returning to the life we dreamed we would have together.

From the day he was diagnosed, the silent message from God, to devote my life to caring for My Love, screamed at me once again. God prepared me to handle this, previously as support to my mom after her almost fatal aneurysm at age 58, followed by brain surgery, with short-term memory loss for six months, and ultimately, her sudden death fourteen years later.

SECTION 2 - DOCTORS & MEMORY LOSS

The paramedics carefully lifted Mark out of bed onto the stretcher. I followed them to the front door, then quickly locked the door. I don't remember the sound of the siren as the ambulance took Mark away to the hospital. My mind in overdrive suddenly grabbed keys, purse, and Mark's wallet, then out to the door in the dark, and drove to the emergency.

When I arrived at the hospital, they wheeled him in. I checked in at the receiving station and gave the attendants the necessary insurance information. I stood at the counter and hoped they would call me back soon. Almost as if time stood still. The only noise I heard was the voices in my head: What does this all mean? Will he be paralyzed? Will he walk again? I need to be with him.

They called me, and I went to Mark in the hallway, until an area was available. After waiting, we moved into a draped, partitioned area. The emergency doctor, nurses, and technicians began a series of x-rays of his stomach area, blood analysis, urine specimen through his nostrils, and CT scan of his head.

While I awaited results, I called his brother, Robert, his sister, Pauline, and my daughter, Ann. Since his daughters were five hours away, I waited to call them until I knew more. The hospital staff gave him morphine medication to relieve his pain. It didn't help, so they gave him another dose. The emergency doctor came in. He was a short man with flush cheeks and told us every test came back normal. The doctor found nothing, and consequently, if Mark stood up alone, he'd be discharged. Only with our help, Mark stood, but very wobbly and not our Mark.

I didn't give. I pleaded and fought for both of us. "My husband is not the same man. Something is wrong; you need to do more analysis to see what is causing his pain. Yesterday, he could walk. Something is wrong."

"It's not as simple as that. With the new hospital standards, the hospitalists, the new name for hospital doctors, are ready to discharge him. They can't find anything in the tests."

"Doctor, I can't accept this. More has to be done."

"I'm sorry. Rules are rules."

"This is unacceptable."

"I can let you have this room for a few minutes more."

SECTION 2 - DOCTORS & MEMORY LOSS

I wanted to break something, shake the doctor by his shoulders until he saw reason, but I kept control. "I need to call his family."

After my discussions with our hospital nurse, Robert, and Pauline, I told the hospitalist that I'd challenge their decision, and I wanted them to keep Mark in the hospital for further investigation of his condition. He was not the same. He walked before. Due to the new medical care provisions, Robert and I were told his case would be reviewed and approved by the medical staff board before admitting him for further testing.

"His case would go before the hospital board for review? Are you kidding me?" I exclaimed.

The hospitalist came in after several hours and told us votes were cast, and Mark was admitted. Due to his altered mental state, I was with him every night. I was never offered any assistance from the hospital for him at night. The family came to relieve me for a drive home to take a quick shower each morning, letting my hair hang dry, no makeup, and back to the hospital. I didn't want to miss the doctor's visit and never knew his arrival time. Never a set appointment time, we were entirely at the doctor's mercy. I often stepped outside of myself, running too fast to morph into the loving, sweet woman I used to be, racing beyond the 'new normal' caregiving woman I became in the onslaught of Mark's condition. I was a third person, who lost ground, like I fell flat and stayed there in a movie theatre scene, with no strong men around to help me up. Would I get up left to my own devices? Or would I stay down? Forever.

They checked his blood levels every day and monitored his platelet levels. I didn't even know what platelets were. In the beginning, they were at a level of 153,000. We were told his INR, "International Normal Ratio," should be a certain level to be safe. Mark's level was borderline too low, not safe.

The hospital chalkboard described Mark as a "Fall Risk," by the attending nurse assistant on duty. Consequently, he couldn't get out of bed without the aid and attendance of the hospital staff. When he needed to go to the bathroom, even with help, it was difficult. Often, before nurses' aid arrived, some five or ten minutes later, Mark already went to the bathroom in his bed, and the bed had to be changed. I assisted with his gown and pads or grabbed the portable urinal as needed. The hospital was often short-staffed and didn't get to the room in time.

On his third day, a female physical therapist tried to teach him to use the walker, but he was still very shaky. Mark was a very private man and had never been in the hospital before. He refused any nurse to touch him when the nurses tried to turn him over from side to side. Without me present to calm him down, he became extremely combative, slapped the nurses, and held his sheet down to cover his body. This side of him was not his old self, but the new self, controlled by the internal terrorist disease which had him entirely imprisoned mentally and physically. I spent every night with him.

One night, while I lay on a reclining chair, my temporary bed, right next to Mark, he leaned over to me, smiling and said, "This is such a nice vacation, honey." Very sweet, but a rude, loud awakening of his condition.

After four days, the attending hospitalist walked me into the hallway and told the family and me that Mark necessitated a transfer to a skilled nursing facility. He could no longer be at home.

"Doctor, he's too young to be in skilled nursing. I don't want him to go to skilled nursing. He's been going to an assisted living for Alzheimer's patients for daycare. Could I take him there?" I asked, in somewhat of a fogged denial. I fought for Mark and wanted him to keep his dignity.

"He needs physical therapy and monitoring of blood work. If they can provide those services, he should go there." It was devastating news and I could hardly breathe. He looked at me with compassion. And I wasn't sure what he saw, me on vacation, about to go jet-skiing or parasailing or hiking?

"Thank you; I'll give them a call."

After the doctor left, I looked at my sister-in-law, and she hugged me. I saw signs of his progression and knew I had to transition him, but I didn't know how. I already saw the horrors of what those places looked like, and I couldn't picture it for my Mark. I knew it was time for me to hand over the baton to the team of caregivers, but I couldn't mentally allow the release. I silently prayed, please, dear God, not a skilled nursing facility. Help us with the right decision. Months ago, I didn't know how I would transition him to a permanent assisted care facility. Again, I thought, is this God's grace to help me transition him into assisted care? I wanted him

SECTION 2 - DOCTORS & MEMORY LOSS

home but was pulled entirely apart. The decision was overwhelming. I talked to the family, my support system, Robert, Pauline, and my daughter, Ann. We all concurred I should transition him permanently on the premise of his need for prolonged physical therapy.

After much contemplation, I called Mark's memory care facility. "Can you accommodate Mark with physical therapy and blood work when needed?" I asked.

"Yes, we can." Exactly what I wanted to hear.

Done, Mark was going for physical therapy. Beyond devastating, but at least he wouldn't have to go to a skilled nursing facility. All day, I bit my lips, chewing the inside of my gums. I had a difficult time finding the right words to tell him. I went home, packed some of his clothes and medications.

The drive to the facility was difficult. We saw the facility on the search for Mark's mom in years past. The staff at reception welcomed me with well-rehearsed, slight Stepford smiles. The waiting area offered water, and the ice tea pitcher and cups for anyone thirsty. The reception area was decorated with two French provincial love seats, a dark mahogany coffee table with a dry flower arrangement, and another side table with a sign-in for guests was welcoming.

I was meeting with the marketing director to sign the necessary papers and give a deposit. I sat and waited for her to receive me. I heard a buzzer when the door opened, and she had a Stepford smile. She asked me to follow her to her office. After she explained a few things, she told me each month the cost was approximately $6,000.

"How much?" I asked in disbelief.

"Six-thousand," the elderly woman repeated. Same smile.

I was numb, as though my body was inside somebody else's life. The marketing director gave me a list of items, other than the clothing Mark needed. They provided a hospital bed, which was too short for 6-foot 2-inch Mark. On my list of items required were a longer bed, a TV from home, a living room chair with the ottoman, and a selection of family pictures.

"We encourage the residents to socialize and watch TV with the others in the living area." She looked at me, smiling-smiling.

SECTION 2 - DOCTORS & MEMORY LOSS

"Are you saying he doesn't need a TV? I thought he could watch his own if he didn't like what the others watched."

"Sure, sure, of course. I understand. Bring whatever you need to make him comfortable." She leaned into my shoulder and said sympathetically, as if he were in hospice instead of a memory facility.

After I saw his new room, I arranged, cleaned and dusted. In the meantime, he used the bed available. I ordered a new, longer bed. I contacted his doctor and got new orders for his prescriptions, necessary for the facility to administer any medications. He couldn't even wear his support socks without a prescription. I was told I had to put the socks on Mark myself unless I got a written doctor order. The facility wanted no liability. We signed our lives away and made arrangements for Mark to go to memory care. Correct that. I signed our lives away.

I watched his physical therapist as she asked him to turn and lean to his side, and then push up to sit as she slowly guided and assisted for his daily exercise. She helped him stand with the walker in front of him, while she strapped him with a large leather belt around his waist. She held at the back, placed his hands on the walker, and helped him stand. She told him she would be with him the whole time. Even with her help, it was a slow process. He was shaky. When they returned from walking the hallway, I thought the timing was right to talk to him.

"Mark, you did a great job, but I know how hard that was. The doctor told me you need to continue the physical therapy when the hospital discharges you. I called the assisted living where you've been and you know the people. They can help you with physical therapy. We're lucky they can accommodate you. I'll visit every day." He looked at me and said nothing, taking it all in. Miraculously, I kept it together. I knew how to do it. The marketing director's smile was my sad mirror.

The day Mark was transported by ambulance to his new residence, I went home to an empty house with a hole in my heart and missed him terribly. He wasn't sitting next to me on the love seat. We didn't have our meals on wicker trays, facing our backyard. I needed a break, but there was a huge void. I devoted everything to him.

"Well, this sucks to hell and back," I said to no one.

SECTION 2 - DOCTORS & MEMORY LOSS

The staff advised me to wait a day to see him. Reluctantly, I decided not to visit him that first evening. It was tormenting.

The next day, our new normal began with the ritual of daily visits before lunch and dinner. I learned the safety door code, walked in and said my hellos to the new community. A mix of elderly people became our new friends. Some walked with stuffed animals in their arms, in wheelchairs, in walkers, and others busy with projects in the activities room. The room positioned in the front with windows gave an outside view of the landscape of hydrangeas, roses, and trees. The residents saw incoming visitors parking in front.

Mark spent four days trying to adjust to this new life, not interested in physical therapy and, not forced to participate. He made excuses, ranging from "I'm too tired," to "I don't feel well."

My chosen daily ritual to help him freshen up, I placed a warm, wet face towel and slowly wiped his face and ears. Then I took his socks off, washed his feet, gave him a lotion foot rub and changed his clothes from the night before, including wet Depends.

While Mark was there he wouldn't allow the staff to shower him. We followed his lead most of the time. But as an order from management, the staff couldn't force him to do anything that caused him to become combative.

SECTION 2 - DOCTORS & MEMORY LOSS

SECTION 3 - HOSPITAL & ASSISTED LIVING

Chapter 19: Embedded
[MAY - JUNE 2012]

Banquet tables and chairs set and ready for the "Friends and Family Day." The weekly luncheon was held on Wednesdays and served in the activities room and the hallway for any overflow of family. It was May 2012, and all the residents and their families milled throughout the halls. An aroma of comfort food floated in the air of grandma's cooking, with ham, mashed potatoes, fresh bread, and cookies. It seemed like a party with a guitarist playing and singing by the staff. Afterward, residents lingered for activities.

"Where is the bathroom?" Mark asked the staff with a look of panic. I was later informed.

"Follow me; I'll show you." They directed him to his room. While he washed his hands, he looked into the mirror. I imagine his face blank with confusion and uneasiness.

"Where's my wife? I can't find her."

"Why don't you follow me? We'll look for her together." The caregiver led him into the hallway and through all the halls as he looked from side to side in each room, passing other people but didn't find me. He walked into the kitchen but found no one.

"Mark, why don't we go into the activities room?" She pointed him toward the hallway.

He walked down another hallway toward the loud voices of people talking and laughing in a large room, seated at buffet tables, while they drew and listened to music. Mark walked in, sat down, and asked if he wanted to draw.

"I want to find my wife first. I need to talk to her! Can you help me?" he said with urgency.

"Sure, I'll get your paper and pencils. Then I'll get you the phone." She left and returned later with paper and the phone. I met the lady with a pleasant smile and a sense of authority, named Katrina.

"Jean, Mark asked me to call you. Normally I would distract him, but I thought since this is new to him, you wouldn't mind talking to him." She said.

"Of course, put him on the phone." I was there earlier and went home to rest. My daily visits in the past three weeks were once in the morning and late in the afternoon.

"Let me know after you finish with your wife, will you?" She handed Mark the phone.

"Can you please come to see me? It's been a long day. I don't know why I'm here? What did I do wrong?"

"Honey, I planned on coming back. I'll be there soon; I love you."

When I arrived, I walked him from the activities room into his studio. His eyes were affected by the medication and sunken from lack of sleep. The pressure in my heart squeezed, then smashed to glass, like an awful mammogram. I had to reassure him.

"You did nothing wrong; you did everything right. I love you more every day." I tightly hugged him and said, "In fact, we received an invitation to a black-tie, prom day event here in a few days. The invitation says, "A Hawaiian Theme," dress in black-tie or tropical attire. We're supposed to wear Hawaiian clothes, like on a cruise ship. With music and dancing, you know how much you love to sing and dance. It'll be fun."

I wasn't sure how I could leave him after what he said. I told him I wanted to find him a jacket for the party. We purchased a lightweight, navy blue travel jacket for the Alaskan cruise we almost went on, and I hoped it still fit. He gained a few pounds. Not in the mood to shop for anything, I wore a dressy, floral blouse with a long dark denim blue skirt. It didn't matter, as long as I was there for him.

On the day of the party, I took his jacket, slacks, and a dress shirt and helped him get dressed. Sad though, his coat was a little snug. In spite of it, I told him he looked handsome. At our entry, keepsake photographs were taken, under a trellis of Hawaiian flowers.

Not standing room only, few residents were in wheelchairs, but almost everyone was in attendance. The room decorated with posters and streamers of Hawaiian flowers, ships with portholes, ocean waves, and fish, mostly drawn by the residents, was in party-mode. Ukulele music played in the background. Women wore formal dresses, footed with either tennis shoes,

SECTION 3 - HOSPITAL & ASSISTED LIVING

sandals, or low heels, including socks. The women's hair adorned with glitter brooches and Hawaiian flowers. The men wore suits and tuxedos. It was their party prom night.

We walked in and sat in the chairs placed at the perimeter of the room. It reminded me of high school dances. We watched the parade of residents enter. Pure innocence in the room with the crowd, aged from the sixties to nineties, who smiled and laughed at their black-tie event. Some had stoic faces with stoned-med eyes, and didn't want to miss, yet questioned whether to partake. Flowered wheelchairs rolled in with dressy patients, who danced and sang to the beat of the Hawaiian music. The music and activities ignited the life of all these residents. They danced, smiled, and waved their hands to their beat.

While we kept our laughter underneath our big smiles, Mark and I looked at each other at the crowd, not holding back. An unspoken look in both our eyes revealed this to be contrived. It was a twisted combination of a funny, sad, and memorable time. When I looked at him at that random moment, I saw enough of him to know; he knew what was going on. We laughed and suddenly, I was uneasy and very displaced, I thought he looked that way too, for at that moment we were in sync. This crowd of residents, either ailing from memory loss, mobility, or motor functions, all participated and fought together for a night of fun, forgetting any problems and joining in their elixir, the music.

Dance and music brought these people a sense of new energy as if they had no ailments. It did the same for my aunt, who suddenly danced at a wedding, forgetting her back trouble.

I asked Mark to dance, and he was a little hesitant, but he got up. We walked to the dance floor, a smooth dancer, he held me tight to dance, and snuggled up to me. I couldn't help but let a few tears out but immediately wiped them away before anyone saw. I thought to myself; I don't want this for our last dance.

* * *

SECTION 3 - HOSPITAL & ASSISTED LIVING

Every day I visited Mark, I walked down the cluster, called "The Orange Grove," toward his room and looked at the glass shadow box at the entry of each resident. Each box displayed pictures of the residents' family, and items of interest. I couldn't bring myself to decorate this entry box. It was permanent. This little shadow box of 18 inches long, 12 inches wide and 6 inches deep, threatened me every day. If I did it, he wasn't coming home, still in denial and criminal thinking about doing it.

In the next few weeks in June 2012, I tried to let go of my fear and finally decorated Mark's empty shadow box. I think it took a couple of months to do it with the utmost dignity. Everyone else in the hallway had family pictures and memorabilia. I never wanted to see him there permanently. Too difficult to do. I can't remember which photos I selected. I imagine I chose my favorite picture of him on our vacation, a picture of him sitting on the deck in Oregon wearing his sunglasses. The light hit them just right and captured a sunset reflection onto the sunglasses.

Along with our wedding picture, I surrounded photos of the children and grandchildren. I thought of our wedding day. And I had to feel as I fumbled a photo of Mark and it dropped to the floor, of letting my precious husband go.

I didn't want him to see me arranging things in his shadow box. Over time, I measured and put the items in while he ate lunch or dinner. I scaled to the inch for width, depth, and length. I reduced pictures and inserted objects to stand them on. Finally, I displayed the images, along with his favorite blue ceramic fish. As I hung the family pictures on his wall, I couldn't breathe, and my mouth watered. By the time I finished, my inner cheeks and lips felt raw from chewing them. I wondered if he would even notice it or say anything about it. I never asked for his opinion. I shucked photos and kept photos, re-sorted, shuffled, a short-changed woman with no direction of how to place his displaced life. How was I supposed to work this out? For either of us? I hoped that Mark had no clue what was inside. Or did he?

To me, the shadow box was cubic zirconia, shiny to look at, plastic as recycled bottle caps. I fluffed and arranged an artificial bouquet of paper dolls.

Why?

Mark was clueless. I accepted the shadow box was for me. It shouted at me, waved at me, and glared at me. Others didn't care. At the longest part of our stay, I realized the box was there to help me accept I'd lost my husband in this place of dead air. Everything inside was to give me strength and to help me remember what Mark could no longer grasp. He had two adult daughters. He had grandchildren. Someone had to take care of them, if not literally, then inside the box where their lives shrunk to fit measured perimeters, dulled down to inches, fighting for space.

At the same time, I became an extravagant vandal who snuck around, hid, and waited for the right time to pounce on the box so no one would see me. Was this my acceptance of it? Or my denial? Who was more alive? Those people living outside the box, or those caught on paper, pushing for room inside it? And where was Mark? My beautiful Mark? Not a cold or flu that could be medicated away with rest, meds and the proper diet. There was no cure. Mark, if put to the test, would gaze right through the photos, recognizing no one. The internal terrorist ate his choices, directed him to think, and act the way it wanted him too; it was dark mold and doom inside his body. There was no more family. The terrorist took every single one of us inside and outside the shadow box, including me, captive.

SECTION 3 - HOSPITAL & ASSISTED LIVING

SECTION 3 - HOSPITAL & ASSISTED LIVING

Chapter 20: Prey
[JUNE - JULY 2012]

As sweet and gentle as Mark was, he grew to exist in some type of warped alternate universe in the facility. For two months during June and July 2012, I played the secret keeper of dreams, organized his room, ate with him, adorned his shadow box, changed the photos, hoped one would spark his memory. He rested on his bed while we waited for his daughter, Tammy, to visit. When she arrived, she brought oldies but goodies music; Neil Diamond, Frank Sinatra, and Tony Bennett. Mark's spirits lifted when he saw his children. We listened to the music and sat on the only two chairs in the room, a plaid chair from our living room, and the small tan cloth chair. Startled when Tammy's phone rang, I assumed she would turn it off or let it go to voicemail. Instead, she took the call and responded in short answers as if bound and determined to keep the call private. My stomach started to a roller-coaster. It irked me. What was more important than visiting with her dad?

"That was Mom. I need to go."

Her visit lasted a few minutes. "Is she okay?" A simple question I asked. You would have thought I pried.

"Mom said my visit was long enough. She wants me to return to relieve her from babysitting Jill's kids." She picked up her purse.

"I love you, Dad." She said as she hugged him. I stood up and walked her into the hallway.

While blood pulsed my temples, I said, "Too bad you have to leave so soon. Thanks for coming." I wondered if Mark was upset underneath his stoic demeanor. We hugged, and Tammy left.

She left the music, maybe proof she visited.

In the interim, Mark's oldest daughter Jill had twins and sent pictures via text. I printed and framed them across from Mark's bed. Assumed, by even me, that Mark wouldn't remember the pregnancy or the delivery, he surprised one of the nurses at the facility. The nurse later told me, "I told Mark the twins were adorable." You couldn't miss the new pictures of the babies, framed in silver ovals, in contrast to the black-framed photos of Mark's family. The babies had matching outfits, one in yellow and the other in green, corn, and peas.

The nurse grabbed my arm. "Listen to what he said."

"What did Mark say?" I said.

"Yes, the twins are cute, if I ever get to see them."

I was shocked. Mark kept some things in his memory bank; the internal terrorist couldn't snuff out his heart. Did his heart sense things his brain no longer registered or identified? Even though his mind barely functioned, was his heart the true sensor of his internal self? Had I looked too long at his eyes to forget his pure, unchanged heart wouldn't give way to an internal terrorist? I looked at Mark up and down, all around, stared through him, possibly in the entirely wrong way. Just as he sometimes stared through me. We needed to laugh. We needed to watch silly movies. We needed above all, to continue to be a husband and wife and a fearless team. Together we conquered! But intrusions of a different sort interfered, attempted to pull apart what was rock solid. So started our journey with the Stepford Wives of Memory Loss Lane.

* * *

At the facility, always a jolt to witness the antics and random visits of the women patients in residence, who thought Mark was their target or prey. I called them Stepford Wives of Memory Loss Lane. These women looked like mature women but were child-like in their actions, innocent and uninhibited. Not uncommon during my visit to see an attractive, dark-haired, plate-faced woman enter Mark's room. Mark's studio bedroom area was divided from the bathroom by an ugly plastic cube-patterned shower curtain, the privacy wall between the living space, the toilet, sink, and overhead mirror. Every time I saw that shower curtain, I made a mental note. Replace butt-ugly shower curtain!

Not uncommon for me to sit in a chair talking to Mark, while he lay on his bed, when the plate-faced brunette walked in, closed his shower curtain, and said, "I'll close for you," and she did with a whoosh.

SECTION 3 - HOSPITAL & ASSISTED LIVING

In their previous worlds, I imagined these women as cleaning fanatics, tidy beyond belief, the superhero women of Scrubbing Bubbles, and liquid bleach.

Another day, a woman who looked like Mark's mom, blonde and tall, walked into his room, while I was in the bathroom, hidden behind the butt-ugly shower curtain.

"Hi honey, let's go for a walk," she said to Mark, not knowing that I was there.

I couldn't see her, but I shocked her with my reply. "Like hell, anybody is going for a walk."

"Oh, no! That's OK," blondie replied and left abruptly as if her toes were on fire.

My daughter Ann, great support to me during this time, worked, so it was hard for her to visit us, but she often called. I usually picked up her calls, as Mark's mind wandered off, and he'd shift into someone who only knew me in bits and pieces, on partial, tainted levels of recognition. The imaginary friends took his attention. Sometimes craving wholeness was essential. Ann saw me whole.

"Mom, you okay?"

"Been better."

"What's going on?"

I stood outside Mark's room, cradling the phone to my ear, pretending it was a warm ray of sunshine. "He's not sure about me, today. I can see suspicion in his gaze. It's hard. Almost every day I have to prove to him I belong here."

"That would be awful."

"It is. Plus, the Stepford Wives."

She laughed. "Watch out for those women. One of them might snatch Mark when you're gone and turn him into a cleaning machine."

Ann was great. She tried to help me. I just felt sick. To be honest, I wasn't sure how long I could keep coming to the facility, afternoon, evening, afternoon-evening and not start to lose it. Everything grew harder to endure or accomplish. I slipped outside of my physical and emotional energy limits, walked a dangerous line between utter exhaustion and

SECTION 3 - HOSPITAL & ASSISTED LIVING

minimal existence. If anyone I knew had been a caregiver, I sought them out. I was too alone to be 'this alone.'

As time moved on, my visits consisted of dinner with Mark. We retired in his room to watch television. As usual, I sat in his chair, and Mark lay on the bed. While he was on the bed, the plate-faced brunette returned, looked at me, and then at Mark. She pointed at him, then said,

"Do you know who that is?"

"Yes, that's Mark, my husband," I said.

"Do you want him?" she asked while she never took her eyes from me.

"Yes, he's my husband, and I love him."

Pause. After walking a few steps, I smiled at her and said, "You go ahead, and I'll catch up with you later."

The lady smiled back and proceeded on. I learned to be passive, not aggressive, or go against what the internal terrorist did to their prey. I went back to my beloved Mark. I couldn't help what happened in this room when I wasn't around. The women at the facility were mostly harmless. Maybe one would even clean his room if we got lucky! Eventually, rather than trying to outrun things at the speed of light, I slowed everything down to a dull walk. Instead of 100 mph, it was 25 mph, less in a makeshift school zone, even less in the area of child-like adults.

Yes, I micromanaged the facility on occasion. Not uncommon for me to find Mark with the same clothes on from the night before.

"Unacceptable," became my mantra.

The staff told me repeatedly, "We can't argue with the resident if they're combative." Mark often was combative when it came to his privacy. Sometimes, he wore someone else's clothes. Previously, at home, on the toilet, he never left the door open. There was no door in his toilet area.

Mark continued to refuse to shower. I didn't blame him. The community shower was in a claustrophobic, stuffy bathroom in the hallway. It was in the hall in a closed-in room with uninvited guests, the caregivers on staff, watching him. Caregivers supposedly checked the resident whereabouts every thirty minutes. He freaked out. Shut down. How much could he take? How much could I take? It wasn't fair. We paid the facility a fortune of six-thousand dollars a month. For that much money, could Mark not

SECTION 3 - HOSPITAL & ASSISTED LIVING

have had ten minutes of private time to shower? It became too much for me to accept. I was furious, and so was Mark.

One day he decided to control his affairs in his way. It was the best he could do. And it backfired badly. I visited early one morning at 9:00 a.m. Upon my arrival, Mark wore his usual signature attire: fave blue baseball hat, long sleeve shirt, fleece jacket, long pants, and laced leather shoes. This time weighted down with three pairs of wet Depends. He was dragging his pants down, with the extra weight of soaking disposable underwear, one on top of the other. I wanted to cry. The ammonia smell was horrible. I knew he peed, probably several times, and the urine gave him a rash. How long was he this way, with three pairs of soaking wet Depends? I was livid and wanted to scream, but kept my cool in front of him. I calmly helped him change his clothes, wiped him, took his three pairs of heavy wet Depends, wrapped them in a newspaper, hurried past the Stepford Wives of Memory Loss Lane, and stormed directly to my new friend, the activities director.

I was volcanic. "This is three pairs of wet Depends that I just took off of Mark. Do you want me to open this for you to see? What would you do if it was your husband?"

The director sat back at her desk, her eyes entirely lackluster as if we were but number two-thousand and one on her 'to do' list. "Take it directly to the staff nurse. The caregivers are under her supervision."

I acted immediately and went directly to the head nurse.

"I just took these three pairs of wet Depends off of Mark!" My hands trembled as I held them up to her.

"I'll take care of it." The nurse replied. She never apologized.

I complained to the executive director, the activities director, and the head nurse in a letter. Again, told the caregivers can't argue with a resident who might become combative. Mark told the caregivers he would change his underwear, but instead, he added another one on top of the existing wet pair. They didn't follow up and check his trash can to make sure he took off the old pair, nor did they take notes to make sure he changed his underwear. They were understaffed and poorly managed by the head nurse.

SECTION 3 - HOSPITAL & ASSISTED LIVING

His one-on-one caregiver didn't call to tell me there were problems. The same day the staff caregiver tried to give him his evening pills and Mark chewed the tablets instead of swallowing them.

The next day, mortified, my gut clenched at the behavior of the facility staff and nurses. I couldn't take my eyes off of them for a second. Thus, I went to visit Mark in the morning. He was wet and not shaved, still in his jeans and nightshirt on the mattress, but no sheets. He didn't want help, and he ripped the name tag off of his one-on-one caregiver. I changed his clothes and took off his nightshirt when I noticed two red marks on his arm where his medical bracelet lay.

"What's this?" I asked Mark. Agitated, he told me the personal caregiver held him down.

Inside I was explosive but again tried not to show it to Mark. I told the caregivers what I found and asked if they knew anything. They accused Mark of hitting the one-on-one caregiver. Also, the new caregiver didn't change or shower Mark, so it wasn't hard for me to dismiss him.

In my extreme agitation, I complained to both executive and activities directors about the incident and continued problems with their inability to monitor his changes and showers. They both offered to help Mark. I suggested they teach the caregivers to place a towel in front of his private areas so that the caregivers could change him with dignity.

The woman activities director offered to help Mark change one morning before the day's activities.

"Here Mark, use this towel in front of you while you change, that way, I won't take your dignity away," she said.

"That's one thing you can't take away from me," Mark replied.

She revealed how he could respond to her remark so quickly, and understand what she said. Mark's heart was alive, vibrant, beating, gathering warrior strength to his soul without apology. "To hell with you all," he would have said, with dignity.

In 2012, Mark experienced the sundowner syndrome, a common side-effect of Alzheimer's, awake late at night until 4 a.m., and slept during the day.

Sundays included church at the facility activities room, the entire room walls decorated with resident designed artwork. We sat in the same seats after the service, but the energy of organ church music changed to lively dance music for the exercise program. The activities director passed out plastic exercise pulleys for the eager participants, including me, to pull the rope around our chairs and legs, for simple and interactive exercises.

Walkers were set around the chairs, next to the wheelchair-bound women and men, who moved around the space. The sound of music filled the air, an electric cord that turned on their magic energy. Alive with their hands moving around, and their faces shined brightly with smiles. Even though I went through the motions, I was in another world, like a foreigner in a strange country. Mark smiled to know I was with him.

* * *

At home later that day, I checked emails. I received an email from Mark's ex-wife to ask me if she could visit Mark. Before I responded, I asked Mark how he felt about it. I didn't think he wanted to talk to her but had to ask him. It was not up to me.

"No!" Did he mean no, or was he considerate of my feelings? I consulted with his brother Robert, sister-in-law Fran, and sister Pauline. We all concurred it was not wise, considering previous situations between the two of them involved drama. She completely changed circumstances to make herself look the best and the center of everything.

I alerted the staff of the possibility of an unannounced visit and asked for a meeting with the executive director. I described his ex-wife's out of control personality and attempts to win at all costs, no matter anyone else's consideration. I took in a copy of her picture as a precaution.

The executive director returned my call. He suggested a meeting with Mark and Robert to ask Mark without me present. Mark's reply to the executive director was: "No, she's a wacko; she has no reason to see me."

The executive director suggested I send his ex-wife an email to tell her Mark didn't want to see her. I tried to respond and express Mark's feelings gently to her, knowing it would cause an eruption. His ex-wife's response confirmed what I expected. "He doesn't know what he's doing. This is between you and me." Evidently, by those words, she wanted a confrontation with me. I let it go and never responded. Everything I was told and read about complicated individuals with an agenda, they love drama. Responding to her would have continued unnecessary and detrimental communication. I didn't allow his ex-wife to be in the center of Mark's environment and new living arrangement transition.

* * *

The next few weeks were especially challenging. Mark barely stayed awake during my daily visits. He kept sundowner hours, awake at night, and slept during the day. It was a challenge to shave his face, clean his scalp and feet, clip his toenails, give him his daily foot massage, and show him my love, sitting with his head drooped over.

The nurse told me Mark called out a profanity to the staff. I was beside myself on what to do; this wasn't him. I didn't know if he would ever adjust to his new life and his new self. I talked to one of the nurses and called the neuropsychologist for advice. The doctor suggested taking him off his regular meds; however, I was afraid of more changes; he was still balancing his blood chemistry, blood values, and INR levels.

It was a problem with changing his clothes, underwear, and showering. A piece of broken glass was found on his carpet. And a water-filled glass with a pill floating inside was on the table. Over the top for me, I marched into the nurse's office and said, "You are the professionals, why aren't you making sure he's changing, taking his pills and showering?"

"He's too difficult. Maybe you can get his doctor to increase his mood meds," they responded. His meds increased. Unfortunately, not only did he sleep through the night, but during the day also. He continued to complain of his leg and back hurting. I thought, should we ever have given him any of their prescribed meds? Not only a lost memory, for all intents and purposes, he became a living breathing medicated zombie.

In some ways, I began to resent life seemed to go on as usual with everyone else. I had my precious daughter, Ann, but I was often alone on the edge of an unpredictable and eroding cliff edge, attempting to walk on the cliff's lip while soil crumbled out from under me. Yes, there were periodic visits, calls, and hugs, but this path toward an Unknown Land was taken by Mark and me alone. No one would follow us. A voice told me to be strong. This inner strength from God gave me a sense of energy, purpose, and caring. I had the freedom to embrace my natural light. The visible transformation of me on the things I used to do daily, mostly trivial things like making sure I had makeup on, no longer important. Yet, I heard my sweet mother's voice. Jean! You need color, put more rouge on your cheeks.

During this time, Mark's daughters called, but the timing was off. When a return call was made to them, in an attempt to do a FaceTime call, he was either in activities or they were tending to their children. I left the home that day and went to church. I knelt. Lighting candles was always a cleansing, to smell the incense and say a few silent prayers in the presence of God's sanctuary.

The next day I awakened at 6:00 a.m. with a telephone call from the staff at the facility. Mark fell, and an ambulance called. Fortunately, I lived only five minutes away. I quickly threw on jeans, a t-shirt, and tennis shoes, hopefully, arrive before the ambulance. Mark was alert and happy to see me.

I said, "How are you feeling, baby?"

His lips barely moved. "Okay."

While we waited for the ambulance, I quickly grabbed things he might need. Razor, comb, clean clothes, shoes, and socks were swiftly thrown into a bag. As soon as the paramedics arrived, they asked, "What happened, how are you feeling?"

"Fine," he said.

When I heard him say fine, my shoulders dropped down. He often complained to me, but in front of the doctor, he would say, "Fine."

They took his vitals, placed him onto the stretcher, and drove him to the hospital. Not easy, but this was the new normal. I followed them. On the way, my mind traveled, and I wondered, Will they find anything this time?

The emergency room only allowed one family member at a time, but I still alerted his family. I looked around the sterile environment with nurses and doctors in a rush, attending to patients. I saw curtains drawn for privacy but heard the nurse or doctors asking questions. As soon as the doctor came in, he introduced himself. He had a calm, sensitive demeanor and was thorough. He said, "I'm Dr. Adams. Tell me what hurts?"

SECTION 3 - HOSPITAL & ASSISTED LIVING

"My knee," Mark said while pointing to his left knee.

"Can you take his INR while we're here?" I asked the doctor. An INR or International Normalized Ratio was used to test how well his blood thinned.

"Yes, we will, but have to wait three hours to do the scans, complications tend to show up later," He said.

We waited three hours for the CAT scans of his head and blood work. The scan showed nothing. The doctor asked me, "Are there any changes?"

"An increase in his mood meds because of changes," I said.

"Falls are more prevalent as Alzheimer's disease progresses."

Another trajectory in the course of this horrible illness, the direction no one wanted. While we waited, I began to run thoughts through my head. I hated Mark was in the facility, away from his real home. I took better care of him. I wanted to do a new budget of what it would cost to bring him home with some assistance. Overwhelmed and unsettled, I discussed my thoughts with the family and talked to the activities director. Everyone appeased me and listened, but they said he was better off at the facility. This time he stayed one full day at the hospital and discharged back to the facility.

The night he was discharged, I followed the transport van to the facility and spent the night with him. I tried to sleep in the chair with the ottoman and watched him until he fell asleep, but he had difficulty.

Not uncommon for Mark to have phlegm in his throat and to spit constantly, but that night there were extra amounts. His throat sounded like he had bubbles in it. I kept getting up to offer a spit-dish. He slept for half-hour intervals, then two-hour intervals. At 10:45 p.m., a caregiver I had never seen came in and said, "Hello Mark, want a bowl of ice cream with whipped cream and chocolate syrup? The show, Friends, is on in the living room, do you want to watch it with us?" The caregiver later showed up in the hallway with a bowl of ice cream and the toppings. I went into the hall.

"I appreciate your kindness, but he has a lot of phlegm. He has reflux and shouldn't be eating dairy or drinking milk," I said.

Mark had difficulty getting out of bed, so I called the caregivers for help.

SECTION 3 - HOSPITAL & ASSISTED LIVING

The next morning when he woke, he needed the help of three caregivers to help get him off the bed. His back still hurt badly; he said, "My back." I kept thinking: How can this be? He just came back from the hospital. I stayed for part of the day until he got up for breakfast, his favorite meal. I took a break to see my daughter, Ann. It was Ann's birthday the next day, so I left to take her a birthday card and donuts. Not much of a celebration time for me, but I tried to go through the motions.

Much younger than most spouses faced with this illness, it wore on me physically and mentally. I fought to control my real feelings and kept a front I was ok.

I went back to check on him and asked the nurse for help to take him to the toilet and change his clothes. I wanted the nurse aware of his back in case he needed more meds. Already on pain patches, sometimes additional Tylenol helped. One time they forgot to date his pain patch, and I noticed it in the same place on his back as the day before.

I often called the caregivers if I didn't return in the evenings to request that they tell Mark I loved him, and I hoped they did. The lack of sufficient caregivers revealed inconsistencies of the care and the changing of the guard among the caregivers who worked part-time. These caregivers, for the most part, were very sweet. I didn't blame them. The facility was short-staffed.

I told Mark I was going home to shower and would be back later. His reply, "That's ok, we'll have a fire later." It was in the summer at 100-degree weather, but ok with me, it was something we always enjoyed in the winter.

Mark's pattern continued to wake late at night and sleep late in the morning. I went every day until I arrived one morning to help him out of bed. He was still in bed.

"Can I help you out of bed? Can you move to this side so that I can help you? I asked.

"You are a whore!" he said while he grabbed my arm tight and tried to twist it, with an awful possessed look on his eyes, he was still physically strong, but it wasn't my husband who spoke. I was in trouble.

It was at that defining moment that I broke free and called for help from the nurses and proceeded to leave, stumbling, lurching, sobbing quietly, desperate to run away from my husband.

SECTION 3 - HOSPITAL & ASSISTED LIVING

Chapter 21: Revealing Moments
[JULY 2012]

I had never been called a whore. It broke me as if repetition or logic of facts somehow made me stronger. My heart ripped from my chest, zapping my body. The disease controlled him. It sucked. I went directly to the nurse's office and could barely talk; I must have sounded like a war victim, a blabbering mess of nerves and emotions. While the nurse was nice, she'd seen it all before. A thousand times. She nodded when appropriate and continued to fill out a file on her desk. "I know. It's awful. I'm so sorry." What else could she say? I was but another shell-shocked wife on the verge of losing it. Ho-hum in her day of extremes that lived on the ripped open side of sanity. She suggested I go home and take a break.

I made an appointment with the doctor for X-rays to recheck Mark's back. Exhausted on top of demoralized to manage his case, coordinate doctor appointments, advocate or beg like a whipped puppy for Mark when all else failed, and few listened. The results; negative.

Everything became more real and difficult to swallow. How could Mark keep going? How could I keep going? The internal terrorist kidnapped and shackled us both. It was July 2012, and Mark had been in assisted living for three months.

A few days later, I received a call from Jill, Mark's oldest daughter. She'd inherited her father's love of photography. Her father's will said his photo equipment went to her. She wanted to look at his gear to see what she should buy in the future. Since his brother was co-trustee of Mark's estate, I discussed it with him to get his approval. Robert concurred it was fine. As fine as it was, it bothered me. Why should I have to do the distribution of Mark's precious possessions already? I drafted papers and Jill signed and dated, she took custody early. Vultures to mind, circling the frail rabbit on the road. My thoughts were not fair to Jill or Mark necessarily - He gave her his camera equipment-but it seemed obscene if not downright ugly to me. I was losing my husband. I wasn't ready.

SECTION 3 - HOSPITAL & ASSISTED LIVING

Rightly so and wrongly so, his things were going to new homes, bequeathed to relatives and stored for later days, away from the light, from him, and from me. My gut clenched and fisted, was a huge knot factory.

The day I arranged for Jill to pick up the equipment, she visited her dad. Out of convenience, I asked her if she wanted to take the artwork on the wall that her dad willed to her, but she declined, only to take the photography gear and books.

That next day, a wreck and a self-acknowledged stalker, I visited Mark three times. The last time at 8:00 p.m. Upon my unanticipated night visit, I didn't see him in his room. I began to look at the adjoining neighborhood clusters of studios and found Mark in another living room, The Peach Orchard unit, watching TV. He walked over without his walker. When I saw him, I told him I would return in a jiffy and left for his walker. I escorted him to his cluster of rooms. We sat in the living room on a cloth sofa, with a round table, chairs, and several patterned cloth armchairs, just like you'd see at grandma's house.

A few minutes later, doll-faced, dark-haired, attractive woman, dressed in her nightgown, tennis shoes, and socks that were secure on her feet as if she were about to take off at any second, came in and sat next to me. Her rigid body language and stares went right through me as if telepathically, she yelled without excuse. You are in my territory, bitch!

On previous days, this same lady circled Mark's room uninvited. This evening she moved around that sitting room, sat in three different chairs, stared right through me with her dark eyes and silently told me I wasn't supposed to be there. I tried to smile at her, as shivers went up and down my back. What happened with the Stepford Wives of Memory Loss Lane when I wasn't around? She staked her claim on Mark, flaunted her power and control as if I even had a chance with him. I was beside myself. She seemed to accuse me without actually opening her mouth or pointing a finger, "So you're the other woman!"

That night the living room overflowed, a catwalk of nightgowns, stares, and musical chairs. The vibes chilled my veins. My rational internal voice told me to leave and let Mark adjust, but my emotional side not ready to give him up to this new world and the raisin-eyed hussies circling the roost. Most of these ladies (and some men) were old enough to be his

SECTION 3 - HOSPITAL & ASSISTED LIVING

parents. After the name-calling from Mark, I tried to transition from the visits to every other day. It was hard. The staff suggested that I wean away with fewer visits, a better adjustment for Mark and me.

AWOL, I thought. The caregiver wanted me to go AWOL and pretend all was okay. The problem was, no one, including Mark, cared if I was there or not. The only one who did care was the dark-haired hussy doll who wanted Mark for herself!

All I could stand was to stay away for one day. I went to have dinner with him, but he was already in the dining room with his table of four. I waited in his room for 45 minutes until he finished. He sat with the older, always smiling, white-haired woman, Pam. I joined them and began a conversation with her, doing my best to keep it light. I admit a desire to throw her across the room. It came to me that I wasn't as nice as everyone said. Pam kept calling Mark by the name Richard. Great I thought. I'll be Elizabeth. Richard Burton and Elizabeth Taylor.

"How long have you lived in your community?" she asked me.

"A good friend introduced me to Mark on a blind date," I said. Mark and I have been together for 15 years and married for 12 years." Then, I shared a funny story about dancing with Mark.

"Richard, we took dancing lessons, didn't we?" Pam said while she turned and looked at Mark. Pam was oblivious to anything I said. I glanced at Mark, prayed for him to support and reiterate my story, and he didn't say anything, I wanted to cry.

"Mark let's go for a walk," I half asked, half suggested.

Pam smiled and said to Mark, "Go ahead, honey, I'll see you later." He stared into the lady's eyes in a trance as if he'd known her his entire life, and trusted her implicitly. Then he asked me for help with his walker, and I proceeded to help him. Later, in his room, he looked at me apologetically.

"I don't ever want to hurt you," he said. It was another revealing moment.

"I know. I'll always love you and never leave you. You can't help what happens sometimes; it's the disease; it's not your fault." I said. Whore! I thought. I wanted to accuse him, yell and scream at him to stop being so mean and an idiot. Wake up! Wake up! Wake up! My emotions were titanic in proportion, upheaved, and turned my spirit upside down.

Mark was in a good mood the next day. 'Friends and Family Day' luncheon was special at the facility. When I arrived, he was in the hallway, smiling and all cleaned up. We sat and had a nice time. Doing better, inhaling and exhaling, trying not to hold my breath, I think I might have even laughed at someone's joke.

Then Mark said, "My back. It hurts."

I took him to his room to lie down. Before I left, the activities director, Katrina, asked me to come by her office. I couldn't imagine why she wanted to talk. Surely, they wouldn't suggest I visit less often. How could they? I was a little shaky when I entered her office, and I couldn't relax. We both stood for a bit. I looked around the small and tidy office, full of books, CDs, and lots of pictures on the walls. A black & white little dog sat on her chair, like on a throne barking authority.

"Sit down, Jean," she said.

I sat. Katrina put the dog on the floor and sat on her desk chair. She looked at papers on her desk and sighed heavily. Crap, I thought. I didn't know what to think as she got up, walked past me, and closed the door. Holy crap. I'm screwed, or we're screwed. Which one is it?

Katrina readjusted her seat at the desk. Polite but blunt, she said, "I'm sorry I have to tell you this, but Mark's friend, Pam, held hands with him." She delivered her message, squint-eyed and dour-faced as if fifty pounds of pressure rode on her shoulders.

I tried to ease her discomfort. "Okay. I don't feel threatened. Mark needs affection. But it makes me sad this is happening. He's so far gone, he doesn't realize what he's doing. He has tried to initiate sex with me while I've been here. That woman looks old enough to be his mother." My voice quivered. My stomach lurched sideways as if I might vomit. At the same time, tears started rolling onto my face. How was this happening to me?

"I admire how you are handling everything. The family wants to talk to you and apologize. Mark isn't her first boyfriend. She had a different boyfriend at the previous facility. She's calling Mark by her old boyfriend's name, Richard. They feel terrible about it." Katrina said.

SECTION 3 - HOSPITAL & ASSISTED LIVING

"I don't want to talk to them. It's not Pam's children's fault. I've noticed some things, so I'm not shocked." I looked down.

"By law, I had to tell you," She dropped her head slightly.

"I'm partly to blame. I told Pam she could hug him when I wasn't here. It's my fault."

"It's not your fault."

"It feels like my fault."

"None of this is your fault."

I looked her bold in the face. "Really? Then why do I feel like I messed up royally?"

The next day, the sky wept along with me. I tried getting in the car, everything outside clouded with rain and inside clouded with tears, and; I couldn't bring myself to visit Mark. I went to lunch with my new girlfriend, Denise, whose husband had Alzheimer's. I confided about what happened with Mark and the hussy/Stepford Wife/Pam. We became close because we shared the same lives, and so alone in our struggles.

Denise and I sat at Starbucks, coffee makers hissing, steam shooting skyward.

Denise said, "My Sam had a lady latch onto him. She thought she was his girlfriend, but Sam knew she wasn't." Denise was adorable, with a pixie-face, and short blonde haircut, she patted my hand through the conversation. We sipped our lattes. For a few seconds, I felt normal.

I went to visit Mark the next day. With my sunglasses on, I greeted him with a kiss. I sat at the lunch table with him and Pam. I wanted to stay incognito so that no one would see my swollen eyes. And I wanted to see how staff and patients, including Mark, reacted if my eyes were covered. My feelings were real, and I wanted to honor them. At the same time, I felt silly; I wasn't Elizabeth Taylor, coveted, and fan-worshipped movie star. And Mark wasn't Richard Burton. It all felt quite delusional and destructive to me. Pride was pride, and I fought for it, staring through dark lenses. My eyes were eggs.

"You look like Miss Cool with your glasses on," Mark said to me.

"My eyes burn." I hoped he wouldn't try to take them off.

In my imagination, smiling, Pam looked sheepish, flushed, caught red-handed, and keenly embarrassed. Why? My woman's intuition on high

SECTION 3 - HOSPITAL & ASSISTED LIVING

alert told me that she did more than hold his hand. My mind went wild. Kissing? Fondling? Sex? I stared her down through my dark glassed perspective. I couldn't help it. Mark was my husband. I could tell by the way he looked at Pam that more happened than a mere handhold. They were vulnerable, but I had hellish feelings of jealousy. They were sick, and at the same time, they kept a secret from me. I asked Mark if he wanted to go for a walk, but he hesitated like he needed Pam's approval first. She made me feel like an outsider and once more like, the other woman. I ground my teeth while my cheeks tightened and my face radiated with heat. I got a hold of myself and wanted to yell, but knew I couldn't.

What would I have shouted? "Screw you all to hell."

After Mark finally got up from the table, I walked him down the hallway. We sat close on a love seat with a view of the patio. I turned and looked directly at him.

"Mark, I know that Pam had a previous boyfriend named Richard at another facility." I waited for him to acknowledge his new name from Pam.

"Boy, you know a lot about her," he said.

"Yes, I do. Remember, I'm your wife, and Pam is a friend." I replied as I held his hand and kissed his fingers.

My new friend Denise, nearby saying hello to others, walked over to visit us. "Hi, Mark, may I talk to you two for a few minutes? I wanted to tell you about my husband, Sam. He had a lady friend, that attached herself to him in the beginning here. Mark, Sam knew what she was doing, but he didn't think of her as his girlfriend. She did, however, believe he was her boyfriend."

Mark said nothing. He just listened with his aloof look. I wondered if he realized what we tried to tell him, or this was so outside of my real world. As hard as this new normal was to accept, I had to swallow it, like chugging on a bottle of liquid Drano.

I needed a break from it-them-everything for a night. I decided to meet my girlfriend, Shelly, for dinner. Afterward, I went to my brother-in law's home in a very emotional state. I sat in the living room and confided to him and his wife, Fran, with Pam's latest events They were welcoming and very supportive. Robert, who usually would joke and laugh, had a very

SECTION 3 - HOSPITAL & ASSISTED LIVING

serious and empathetic face, and Fran, always sweet and endearing, walked over to hug me.

That evening I had another sleepless night, while I imagined catching the two lovers in a locked embrace. Ridiculous as it seemed, it was real, and it was agonizing. I took another melatonin around 2:47 a.m. I tossed and turned the remainder of the night until I finally got up. After my morning routine pee-brush teeth-pull hair out of my face, I looked in the mirror and thought I appeared at least ten years older, with bags and dark circles under my eyes. I was 20 pounds heavier. I didn't watch my diet since his diagnosis, not a lucky one who didn't eat during stress. I was the opposite; I loved bread and other carbs, especially ice cream. I began to have a glass of wine every night to help me sleep. All that added to my weight and my lack of exercise at the gym.

That Sunday was the middle of summer, but I needed some exercise, so I walked the fifteen-minute walk to visit Mark that morning. In the path of the busy street, I heard the birds singing; and the sun warmed my face, as though it was God's light and love shooting through me. A good reminder, I wasn't alone on this journey. I needed His love to keep me centered.

Each time I entered the locked-down facility, the girls at the desk were cheerful. Most times, Mark, my favorite person, smiled, but this morning fragile, sleeping at ten in the morning so innocently, completely consumed by the internal terrorist. His poor feet, hung from the side of the bed, like elongated bats hanging upside down. His jacket still zipped on, with pants soaked at his pelvis. I walked to the hallway and asked for help from the caregivers. They were always helpful, sometimes out of breath, needing more time, but available.

Clean up on AISLE TWO! I thought unable to help make miserable jokes.

On Sunday, around 10:30 a.m., the caregivers combed and styled-the ladies' hair in the hallway, and men sat at the table or on the sofa reading the newspaper or watching TV. The caregiver helped to change his pants and got him ready. While I washed his eyeglasses and shaved him with the electric razor, Mark made horrible faces with a thunderous attitude, as if we tortured him. The caregiver proceeded to wipe his buttocks. I tried to

SECTION 3 - HOSPITAL & ASSISTED LIVING

calm and soothe him. "It's okay Mark, everything will be fine. We just don't want you to burn and hurt." It was the same tone I used with my daughter when I tried to stay calm and in control. Not always the case, I wasn't perfect, frustrated at times, and yelled at the top of my lungs.

I took him mandarin oranges and an energy bar. Afterward, I offered to him, but he declined. His brother and sister-in-law knocked at the door.

"Good morning! Your girls are coming to visit this morning," Fran said. She gave me another fabulous hug. "They've been on vacation for a week. They'll stop by on their way home from the lake. How ya doing, Mark?" Fran asked.

"Fine," he said.

After the church service, I suggested breakfast outside the facility, Denny's, or IHOP. Mark's eyes perked up. Fran suggested only breakfast because of time constraints. I agreed, so we got Mark ready to leave, grabbed his walker and began the trip to the car. I couldn't wait to go out in public with him again, hold his hand, kiss his cheek, watch as he ate bacon and eggs. I was in for another rude awakening and fact about Alzheimer's. Mark's idea of 'his home' had shifted and solidified.

In almost four months, this facility became Mark's new home. Each time we left for an outside excursion like eating out at a restaurant, it was a difficult task. Even though he had been to this exact Denny's in Fresno many times before he got sick, it was all unfamiliar to him. He got confused when we walked up to the restaurant door. He looked down at the ground, it wasn't the solid color of the carpet at the facility. The sidewalk had indentations and lines, and the restaurant courtyard floor was uneven with bumpy tiles. The patio tables and chairs too close together, made him shaky and he lost his balance. I thought, is this a mistake? Another mistake in a long line of mistakes around anything to do with hope and being normal with Mark?

After we got settled inside a booth, Mark became his old self in some ways, a great conversationalist. He bantered with his brother, with jokes going back and forth and lots of laughter. They reminisced of the time Mark came home late, whistling in the hallway after winning a twist contest at the D` Markee. It was a sneak back to the past, which at times happened, the random ins and outs of Alzheimer's disease. Did the smell of breakfast, bacon, eggs, toast, and potatoes in the air help? Or was it sitting in the safety of a booth we previously sat to have lunch or dinner? Afterward, we went back to the home to prepare for his anticipation to see his kids.

His kids came later. He sat on the living room chair, with all four grandkids sitting on each of his legs and the chair arms. He loved his grandchildren. I loved my grandchildren. It was a magical moment.

"Are you pretty?" He asked his granddaughters.

"Yes," they said while they giggled.

"How's your baseball doing?" He asked the oldest grandchild.

"Good Grandpa," he replied.

The youngest grandson looked just like pictures of Mark as a child. Mark went through all the motions of being a grandpa. He lit up and was over the top, while he laughed and smiled with them in his arms. He enjoyed the kids, but I don't think he remembered all the grandchildren's names.

"It was good to see you, I enjoyed our time," Mark said to me.

"So, did I," I said, thinking it was for a sneaked second, back to old times.

"I love you," he said.

"I'll always love you," I replied.

"Do you know why you are here?" I hesitantly asked.

"No," he said.

"It's because of your illness. You know how your feet, ankles, and legs are swollen, that's why. I miss you every day, but we will get through this." I said as I hugged him.

I reminded him to sleep in his bed with his legs elevated and not to fall asleep in the chair or sofa, my daily mantra to him before I departed, sometimes teary-eyed, sometimes devastated. I went home and texted his daughters to tell them how much their dad enjoyed their visit and thanked them for coming.

I met all of Mark's family on another Wednesday for 'Friends and Family Day,' along with Robert, Fran, Pauline, and his favorite cousins from the foothills. They received a phone call about Mark's illness and drove down to give support. Music serenaded the residents and their families, but

Mark wasn't there. I began to search for him, walked toward his room and saw him in the hallway, while he attempted to walk with Pam holding onto his walker. I tried to be cheerful as I approached them and walked him into the luncheon area. Pam saw me and walked toward her family table.

All the banquet tables set, residents and their families were seated. It was very festive with the staff playing guitars and singing along with the families. I had a nice visit with Mark, however, Pam sent me bad energy vibes (The other woman whore!), and ignored me but later tried to get Mark to walk her back to her room. It was out of my control. I had to ignore Pam and let go of her actions. Perhaps if I knew her before her horrible illness, things might have been different, but trying to assess what to react to around her motivations and what to dismiss as harmless, took its toll on me. I dug for my 'better self' and kept digging.

When I walked him into his room, I noticed there was a Tylenol pill on his floor. My face heated up, and my chest tightened, evidence the caregivers didn't confirm that Mark had taken his medication. It was unacceptable and careless. I grabbed the pill and stormed into the kitchen to make them aware of their mistake. With a frown on my face and a look of anger, I asked all the caregivers on duty. No one owned up to the error. I was sure they were sick of anyone, including me, micromanaging their work, but I didn't care. I knew they were understaffed. Each resident accounted for every thirty minutes on a shotgun approach, going in all directions to answer a button call if someone yelled for help.

I went home that day and rested before I met his out-of-town cousins, Robert, Fran, and Pauline, for dinner. The conversation kept light, but the undercurrent, beneath their smiles and jokes, made me aware they were cautious of the serious nature of our escalating situation.

I met these cousins about 15 years before. They were kind to tell me I was responsible for helping Mark find his 'fun buttons' again, to help him reclaim the spirit of fun he had before his first marriage. They told me he lost himself, surviving a marriage that to him was soul-crushing. He'd stayed married for approximately 25+ years for the sake of the kids. These cousins on his dad's side of the family were lively and full of fun. I wanted to hug them. For the first time in a long while, people actually saw me as empowered, rather than victimized. I wasn't 'the other woman.' I was The

SECTION 3 - HOSPITAL & ASSISTED LIVING

Woman. Marks' Woman. And I was damned proud of it. Mark was my hero. My angel. My light.

* * *

I decided to call Mark and check on him after dinner.

His caregiver said he slept with his legs hanging over the side of the bed. So frustrating, why couldn't they help him with his legs? I gave them the benefit, thinking, maybe they were afraid he would awaken and startled, hit them. I asked, "Can you please help him elevate his legs?"

"Sure, I will." The caregiver said.

He had not seen his daughters this month, before his cousins came to visit on Wednesday, 7/25/12. It was timely that his favorite cousins came to visit him on that Wednesday for, 'Friends and Family Day.'

At the beginning of that year, he was introduced and transitioned part-time, a few days of the week, to enjoy the social activities at the facility. Sometimes he enjoyed it; other times he needed an escort from the car to the inside. He didn't want to be without me. As much as I loved him, I needed my sanity back, even if just running errands. I feared he might wander off and get lost. It was a new, unnatural consideration and care I had for him. I was not his mother, but his love. Still, he needed to be cared for as a child, looked every bit as an adult, but vulnerable like a child. He didn't look like the same happy smiling-faced guy, with the quick-witted humor, but stressed stoic eyes, weary from the medication.

* * *

It was as though a convergence of Angels surrounded us, and followed the realigning order of God's plan to prepare all of the family for Mark's readiness for the best to come and the worst to follow. That is, the best for Mark and the worst for the family.

SECTION 3 - HOSPITAL & ASSISTED LIVING

SECTION 3 - HOSPITAL & ASSISTED LIVING

Chapter 22: 4th Trip to the Hospital
[JULY 2012]

The next day, Thursday at 8:30 a.m. on July 26, 2012, the nurse called from the assisted living facility, Mark didn't feel well and refused breakfast, his favorite meal. Apparent his pain patches weren't working. I rushed to the facility, while he lay on his bed, still in his clothes from the night before, a t-shirt, underneath a long sleeve shirt, with his favorite zippered fleece jacket, baseball hat, and wet pants, and a scruffy beard. Not uncommon to find him this way.

"Where do you hurt?" I asked.

"Back and neck." He lay still.

I hugged and kissed him and told him I'd return quickly. I asked the caregiver to help remove his soiled pants because I couldn't lift him. I didn't want to move him the wrong way. He didn't move his face, a very different day, marked with stress lines around his eyes. I was queasy like I wanted to throw up, while a chill went up to my spine like ice fingers. Immediately, I asked for a Tylenol for him and knelt by the bed. A half-hour went by, but no relief.

"Do you feel like eating anything, maybe a sandwich and juice?" I asked him.

"Okay," he said.

I walked out and requested the snacks from the caregiver. He slowly took a few bites of the sandwich, but he didn't want it. I called the nurse and asked her to check him. She took his vitals, and they were okay, but something was wrong. I was beside myself. I didn't know what to do, as his back and neck were chronic problems.

"He had the Tylenol this morning, and they haven't helped," I said to the nurse.

The nurse snapped, "He can't have another Tylenol until 3:00 this afternoon."

"He's in pain, what else can you give to relieve him?" I wanted answers from her. In my mind, something was going on, something's wrong. On top of his back pain, his ankles still swollen.

"I'm not a doctor; maybe we should call an ambulance," she said.

"Yes, call one. I'm upset; the girls still don't make sure to elevate his legs."

"It's hard when he won't let us elevate his legs," the nurse argued.

I wasn't in the mood to debate, but he had already been to the hospital three times in the last three months, and they found nothing wrong on the X-rays. While we waited, I knelt next to the bed, leaned over and held him in my arms, and said, "I love you more and more every day. Honey, this is in God's hands, let's pray." There were days when I was lost and questioned things, and then suddenly, I felt peaceful. My faith in God never failed me, he was with us every step of the way, and he stewarded me to help in my devotion to my husband.

"God, we trust that you'll guide us through this time," I said, and Mark grabbed my hand and held on.

The paramedics arrived, took his vitals, and put him on the gurney to take him for the fourth time in four months. I watched them roll out my exhausted, severely pained husband. I questioned how this could be happening to us? Excuse me, Mark was the one tortured, not me. I should have felt like kicking the furniture, screaming and yelling, but instead, and even though I was somewhat lost, there was an unbelievable veil of calm over me.

When they left, I went through the motions and pulled things together, a set of clean clothes, shoes, comb, and an electric razor, not knowing what was in store.

We'd left for the ER the first time from home, and then two more times from the facility. I called his brother, sister, his daughters, and my daughter to let them know. I went directly to the hospital. When I walked into the emergency room, again with a full waiting room, I went to the counter and listened to all the busy attendants.

"My husband was just brought in. He has Alzheimer's disease, and he'll panic if I'm not with him."

"Ma'am, we can't let you go back. The hallways are full of patients waiting for the exam area. I'll call you as soon as I can." The attendant smiled and seemed well suited and acclimated to his job, turned away from me.

I pleaded. "The staff let me go the last three times in the last three months."

"Ma'am, I can't let you go now." My shoulders dropped, and I reluctantly went to the waiting area.

Unlike the first three times, the emergency room didn't allow me to stay with him until he was moved into a room. I panicked, and couldn't sit still knowing Mark was uneasy without me, and with all the other sick patients. We arrived at the hospital emergency at approximately 10:00 that morning.

While I waited, I took a seat. Distracted for a few moments of relief, I saw a woman holding her innocent baby girl with an adorable squashed up face against her mom's shoulder. Her rosy cheeks pressed up tight underneath a lacy cap on her head. Socks inside her gold ballet shoes matched her sweater. This darling little angel was in the middle of the craziness with sick people, but illness doesn't discriminate and brings surprises. Waiting rooms in the hospital can be very unsettling. I was there among other ill patients who waited for themselves or one of their loved ones. At 11:30 a.m., they placed him in another hallway with a curtain pulled around him for privacy. I was finally allowed to join him. I walked down the two halls, where Mark's gurney was aligned parallel to other patients in the same hallway, I wondered what exposure we had with all the other sick patients.

When the doctor finally came, he opened the curtains and tried to examine Mark. Still, in the open hallway, Mark reacted was combative, and pushed them away. He never got over being cattle-called into the emergency hallway. I didn't blame him.

"No, leave me alone!" he yelled and pushed their hands away. He had never been to a hospital before his first visit four months ago.

"He has no privacy here in this hallway!" I yelled at the doctor.

"He did this last time he was here." A young, inexperienced nurse commented without any empathy. She said it in front of Mark, and then I realized she didn't know how to handle him properly.

"There's no privacy in this hallway, and you expect him not to react in front of total strangers?" I said furiously.

SECTION 3 - HOSPITAL & ASSISTED LIVING

The same attending doctor examined Mark four months ago, who wanted to discharge him because he couldn't find anything wrong.

"Nurse, let's move him to that area," the doctor said, while he pointed to an area between two other areas, away from the middle of the hallway, blocked and in a more private space, in between two other draped areas.

Once they moved him, the doctor examined Mark in an emergency-designated space, also draped around him. The doctor walked away. In that new space, Mark was lucky to have a very empathetic group of nurses and technicians. While the nurse started a chart and took his vitals, I expressed my disgust.

"I need to tell you; we just had a bad experience. A young, unsympathetic, inexperienced nurse doesn't know how to keep her mouth shut in front of my husband," I said.

"I'll make sure to say something about it." The new nurse said with compassion.

The next nurse came in and asked me questions about the chain of events. There were three attendants in our little space, giving Mark their full attention.

"When did it start? How's he feeling?" She asked.

"My husband's been in excruciating pain. His symptoms are the same ones that brought him to the hospital the first time in April, four months ago," I said.

"We will be taking X-rays of his back and neck. Do you think he will be able to get on a straight board?" she asked, looking at me with concern.

"I don't think so. He's been in a lot of pain. He couldn't lift his neck or anything before we came to the hospital."

After the X-rays, a CAT scan, and a test of his mucus, they found bacteria. He was admitted to the hospital around 11:30 p.m. They put him on an antibiotic and monitored his temperature.

The doctor came in later, with an attending nurse and informed us, "Mark has bacterial bilateral pneumonia."

"Doctor, what about the chest X-ray Mark had the first time? How long has he had pneumonia? Is it because of his asthma susceptibility? Has the reflux problem caused the infection?" This had been wearing on us. My heart pounded fast, and I wanted answers.

SECTION 3 - HOSPITAL & ASSISTED LIVING

"The infection might take two months to heal. Mark needs a liquid breakfast, so we can see how he swallows. The food at dinner has to be a thick soup and with only ice chips. I'll be in later to see how he's doing." The doctor never responded to my questions.

The nurse asked me, "Do you want a sitter for Mark tonight?"

"Yes, the other three times I've been here, no one offered it. I stayed with him every night and slept on a reclining chair."

Later that day, the hospitalist doctor came to see Mark. He said, "If he continues to have the problem, you'll have to feed him with a feeding tube until his Esophagus heals." Feeding tube? That doesn't sound right.

A few years ago, my uncle's hospice nurse told us a feeding tube would prolong the inevitable. Not using a feeding tube would allow a more peaceful death. The complications can fall into four major categories: mechanical, e.g., tube blockage or removal; gastrointestinal, e.g., diarrhea; infectious, e.g., aspiration pneumonia, tube site infection; and metabolic, e.g., re-feeding syndrome, hyperglycemia. The type and frequency of complications arising from tube feeding vary considerably according to the chosen access route, and gastrointestinal complications, without a doubt, the most common.

I took the emergency room nurse's offer and got a sitter for the first night, but I stayed with Mark for part of the evening. I had to get some rest for the next day. This one had been such a long one without much sleep the night before and hardly any food.

The unit coordinator saw me with the sitter and said, "Maybe you don't need the sitter since you're here." I pointed to the hallway and walked out and motioned her to follow me.

"I was here previously four times and had no help for ten days. I need to go home and get some rest. I need help at night. I'll be here until after he eats his dinner. They told me at emergency under these circumstances, a hospital sitter could be provided during the day and especially at night. On Thursday and Friday mornings, they said they had no one available on Saturday." I called the head nurse.

"We are short-handed, but we can all take turns and pitch in for you. The hospital is short-staffed most of the time. We used to be assigned seven patients per nurse assistant, and now we are assigned double. We

SECTION 3 - HOSPITAL & ASSISTED LIVING

have not found anyone for tonight, but we'll take turns, and make sure someone is here. Don't worry. We'll trade off being here, a half-hour at a time." I couldn't believe how much she revealed a lack of staff. A real wake-up call to hear they were short-staffed. How can I leave Mark alone with this information?

I went into the bathroom. After peeing and while washing my hands, I looked into the mirror, and thought, I don't want to leave, but I'm beyond exhaustion, and I look worse than I feel. Only one night, I just need one night. It was difficult to go home, but I went and got into bed.

That night I received a call from Mark with the nurse's help. "Are you coming back?" Mark asked.

"I'm right here if you need me, Mark, I just need a little sleep, and I'll be back. I love you." I replied. I don't remember falling asleep.

The next morning came in a blink. The alarm went off at 5:30. I quickly showered, put on sweats, no makeup, and went back to the hospital.

When I arrived, Mark was on oxygen because he couldn't breathe easily. He had discomfort from the medication and needed relief. He was supposed to have physical therapy that day. I thought, how much more can he take? I didn't know how he would be able to manage it. He wasn't eating much that day and slept a lot throughout the day. I couldn't leave him like that at night, so I arranged for the nurse to bring another bed in his room, and I stayed.

Waiting for the doctor to arrive, it felt like time stood still and didn't move. In stressful times, families rely on and are at the mercy of the doctors. They hope they time it right to be in the room when the doctor arrives for his assessment. There was never a window of time given for their visit.

Since Mark's daughters lived out of town, they tried to assist by telephone. The oldest daughter's suggestion to give her father an Epidural injection for his back pain was rejected by the doctor, no reason given. The youngest daughter said she was coming to see her dad. She later called and had a change of plans and didn't say why. I left her a voicemail and asked what her plans were, and when would she be available for a phone call. Her return call was a reply on voicemail, "I'll be home from 11:30 on. What are the numbers indicated on my dad's oxygen tank?" She studied nursing and said there were numbers on the machine that meant something.

SECTION 3 - HOSPITAL & ASSISTED LIVING

My message: "I can't read it. Tammy, I need you here. There are too many numbers to read."

A physical therapy aid came in and told me that Mark should be at 95 degrees when he eats and 15 minutes after. A friend's husband, a gastroenterologist, said Mark should be sleeping at 45 degrees, not on pillows, but elevated by a hospital bed, or he would continue to have problems with respiration pneumonia.

Another doctor called a hospitalist, who was tall, overweight, unfriendly, and pale-skinned, finally came in and checked on Mark. He didn't smile. I didn't trust him. After he looked at a few things on his chart and did his once over on Mark, he asked me to follow him in the hallway. I couldn't imagine what else he would drop on us.

"Mark needs skilled nursing. The assisted facility he's in now can't accommodate his needs." He said this like he was talking about a shopping list, hardly gave me eye contact.

"How do we solve Mark's reflux and back pain at the same time?" I asked.

"You solve the most important, the reflux and his needs to keep him elevated, to help prevent pneumonia from continuing or coming back, and continue the meds for his pain."

I didn't get the answer I needed, so I talked to a family friend doctor on staff. He agreed to speak to another doctor about my concern on medication management, so we consulted with the specialist. While we waited, Mark was finally able to talk to his oldest daughter and we tried to call the younger daughter, but she was in San Diego and didn't hear her phone.

Mark was on a thick liquid diet of foods and drinks. The thin liquids complicated his problem. He didn't eat much for lunch that day but did a little better at dinner with soup. He didn't like any of the thick liquid diets, especially, the milk nectar. I didn't force anything on him. I wanted him comfortable and not stressed. He looked so vulnerable in bed with the oxygen tank, needing help for everything. He was stripped of his privacy on an hourly basis, with the nurses periodically checking his pressure, blood, temperature, his wet pads, rearranging his pillows, and moving him from side-to-side to prevent bedsores.

SECTION 3 - HOSPITAL & ASSISTED LIVING

In the meantime, Robert, Pauline, and I went on the hunt for the dreaded skilled nursing facility. Although assisted living communities may have memory care units on the premises, the two types of care are not synonymous. Memory care is a distinct form of long-term skilled nursing that specifically caters to patients with Alzheimer's disease, Dementia, and other types of memory problems. Memory care facilities and areas of skilled nursing have Alzheimer's patients with lockdown areas. The different types of assisted living are:

1. Assisted Living Facility: Patients live independently and manage their food intake with minor assistance required for bathing and dressing. Regular assisted living provides seniors with personal care support, such as meals, bathing and dressing, and medication management.

2. Short Term Care Facility: Patients must have continual monitoring for medications, usually bed-confined, and round-the-clock care.

3. Skilled nursing is a term that refers to a patient's need for care or treatment that can only be done by licensed nurses. Examples of skilled nursing needs include complex-wound dressings, rehabilitation, tube feedings, or rapidly changing health status.

The first one had a one to the two-year waiting period. It was an old, sterile, clean interior environment with nicely landscaped grounds. The next one had a two-year waiting list, but they offered a possible room in the short-stay, for the transition to a long-term facility. The third one, we couldn't see. The last one was an awful, worn building, no one in front to greet you, had a vacancy, and in my opinion, should have been condemned. I would never send my Mark there. We'd seen it previously, on the search for Mark's mom. It screamed of near-death with the stench of urine, drooping heads, stoic looks, and wheelchair patients with utter despair on their stretched faces as if to say, "Take me away from here."

One of Robert's friends, who was at one of the skilled nursing facilities, had the same disease as Mark. He was in a wheelchair, with his eyes closed while being fed, opened at some intervals.

"You have such beautiful blue eyes," I said to him. With that, he opened his eyes completely and smiled and seemed to open his heart.

* * *

SECTION 3 - HOSPITAL & ASSISTED LIVING

Still very drowsy, Mark slept most of that day, so I asked the staff if they could reduce his dosage to see if it worked, to prevent him from being so tired. While we watched him sleep, Robert, Pauline and I discussed the death of a reverend who had cancer. The minister was capable of pre-recording his hour-long eulogy. Mark suddenly opened his eyes from his bed and said: "Get out now!" Even though his eyes were closed, we didn't know he was aware of our conversation. He was slower and distant at times, but still randomly aware.

I felt sick; he'd heard anything about us discussing a funeral. It wasn't fair to him, and I realized we had to be careful about future conversations in front of him, whether he appeared awake or asleep.

The day after, he was more alert and combative with the nurses off and on. So, the nurses called me in to help change him, and when I noticed the oxygen tube was twisted and made him uncomfortable. The staff hadn't seen his oxygen tube was turned by accident. He had every right to be upset.

The next morning, as soon as my brother-in-law, Robert relieved me, I went home, showered quickly and returned before the doctor arrived and before Mark's 11:45 a.m. swallow test assessment.

The hospital attendant pushed him in the wheelchair downstairs for the MRI of his esophagus to watch how he swallowed. I walked along.

"I only want one picture, and I don't want a bird feeder," Mark said to me while we waited his turn for the swallow test. Again, his random awareness of the situation, his translation of the feeding tube. He was present and knew the impact. Amazing, he remembered what the doctor said, but his Alzheimer's brain translated it from feeding tube to a bird feeder.

They gave Mark a few different types of liquid to observe how he swallowed and how long it took for it to go down. The technician looked into my eyes after it was completed, and showed me the video scan of Mark's esophageal muscles as he swallowed. She asked me to follow her into the next room. She spoke quietly and sensitively.

"He has a delayed swallow, due to his altered mental state. His Alzheimer's brain doesn't tell him to swallow. He has to alternate different food textures, and will continue with thick liquid foods but has to alternate with thick lemon water. I will order a speech therapist for his therapy. His

SECTION 3 - HOSPITAL & ASSISTED LIVING

delay is probably from his mental status due to Dementia and Alzheimer's. The brain is not directing him to swallow." After I heard it, my stomach turned and started to cramp. I knew what was coming, the next phase of more serious hurdles to maneuver. I had to keep it from him and only wrap more love on him no matter what happened and above all else to keep him comfortable. Being unable to swallow voluntarily was terrifying.

The days that followed, my Mark, my favorite person, my angel, suddenly, now lost all hostility and was peaceful. It was surreal, precious, beautiful, and heartbreaking too. He'd reached the other side of somewhere I couldn't go. Ever. I asked him to pray with me to God to keep his spirit within him. I knew he did. I could see it on his gentle face radiant with the calm of his new self. He'd come full circle, from peace to battle to peace again. Only with this experience, we understood he wouldn't be coming home with me, ever again.

He only walked once with the physical therapist and stayed mostly in bed. This was a life-changing time, and we all felt it. My few tears were honest and hard to dredge up. I went for lengths of time as dry as a desert sunset. Mark and I understood our impasse. We were at an impossible crossroads, and I wouldn't be traveling with him up his certain path. I would be going a different direction, and eventually, even when we glanced over our shoulders, we would be gone in the distance, no more joined or together in this physical sense and no more in love than we'd ever been. We had to let go of each other.

As Mark and I shared our silent good-byes, I wasn't sure his daughters really understood what was happening to him, or how soon things were changing. One had a weekend spa with girlfriends before she even went to see her dad, because of the stress. His daughters lived five and two hours away, both with small children. One never came this time to the hospital, as she had a change in plans. I know it was tough, but I didn't understand the denials by his daughters of his condition. I knew they desperately loved their dad, but it was probably difficult for them to see their strong dad in a vulnerable place. Simply no rules and no judgments made. Everyone faces a loved one's death in the way they need to. I said a prayer for his daughters. I said a prayer for us.

SECTION 3 - HOSPITAL & ASSISTED LIVING

The hospitalist doctor came into Mark's room later that day and again informed me that Mark should go on a feeding tube so that he could get better nutrition. His bedside manner left me frustrated like I hung from a cliff with no way out but to jump. I hated this hospitalist doctor more than I can write about. But hate doesn't help, and in the long run, I wanted to let negativity and regret float by me on a white water current heading out to sea.

The weight of it made me weak and unable to breathe well. When his brother and sister came in, we walked to the hallway, and I told them. Ann, my loving daughter, and my sister-in-law, Fran, came next, and I went through the story again. Everyone was in horrible quivering shock.

A feeding tube, at least in our minds and hearts, was entirely the first step on Mark's journey to a terminal situation.

There was no acceptable or ready skilled nursing facility available, and the feeding tube decision still questionable. My mind raced. Should I bring him home? Or, what will it cost to have the help needed for him to be in a wheelchair and a feeding tube? I thought of what the doctor said, "If he's to prevent pneumonia from continuing or coming back, he needs to continue the meds and sleep elevated." It was all complicated because of his memory. No one would watch him like I would love him and care for him until the end. No one would stop me. No one would tell me what to do or when to do it. No one would pretend I wasn't his forever wife.

"Mark, do you want the tube?" I asked.

He was so uncomfortable. When someone can't swallow right, it forces the body to undergo enormous stress. He was miserable, unable to shake his head. For my dear Mark, no tube.

I wouldn't put him through it. I remembered the visits with Mark to see my uncle, who was on a feeding tube from ALS before he died. We had both seen him and said it was a horrible way to survive.

Under Mark's health care directive, I was his primary decision-maker for his care. There was a load on my shoulders with the horrible things to think about and decisions that had to be made concerning his care. I consulted with Robert, Pauline, Fran and Ann, who were my main support in town. I talked to his daughters, but ultimately, I was his main caregiver and it was my decision. I wasn't ready to hand the baton to total strangers for the delicate care of his failing condition. Even though I cared for him in the last six years at home, at the same time, I knew I couldn't do it alone.

I prayed to God to help with difficult decisions. I didn't want my Mark to suffer living with a feeding tube and was almost to the edge of my physical and emotional limits. I'd gone without true rest or sleep for months. When I managed to make it to bed at home, I screamed into my pillow. If indeed I did sleep, it was as a wounded shell, my stomach a ball of flame and ash, the knot in my throat, a constant reminder that any day now, I would lose my beloved and he would journey without me and I would have to go into our house and clean it and scrub it and straighten and dust and understand finally, that Mark was a traveler on an adventure and God had him in His arms and Mark was never coming home.

SECTION 3 - HOSPITAL & ASSISTED LIVING

Chapter 23: Angel Discharge Nurse
[JULY 2012]

On our previous visits to the hospital, the discharge nurses offered consultations to the families at the end of patients stay, if their loved ones were not returning home. On July 31, 2012, I walked over to the central nurses' station and requested an appointment with the discharge nurse, and later that day a meeting was set. I wanted to discuss the conversation with the doctor about the feeding tube, our inability to find a suitable skilled nursing facility, and ask for suggestions or alternatives.

I met with the nurse that day, and coincidentally it was the same one who discharged Mark on his first hospital stay. She was middle-aged, blond, had a friendly smile, and looked compassionate. I stood in the hallway near her cubicle, a small counter with a computer between two walls and open to everyone with no privacy. I told her what the doctor suggested to our family. My words came out shaky and fast. I said, "I know my husband doesn't want a feeding tube. I don't want that for him either. Even if there was a space for him in a skilled nursing facility, I don't want him in that kind of environment. I'm beside myself with what I should do." The nurse listened and looked at me with sympathetic eyes.

"In my experience, you are prolonging the inevitable. Due to the progression of your husband's disease, it will be about six months before his death." She spoke with a kind heart and candor. Hearing those words made everything in my body tingle like I was snow globe that someone had shaken. My mouth watered, my head got hot, and I'm sure my face flushed red. I had to pull myself together and calm down. I wanted a meeting with the hospitalist doctor. I was livid. He didn't have the decency to inform me of the real truth of Mark's current condition.

"Your husband could probably qualify for hospice care. You can take him home or to a hospice facility. If you want, I can order an evaluation. Would you like me to?" The discharge nurse said and looked away.

SECTION 3 - HOSPITAL & ASSISTED LIVING

My voice quivered, yet I had to step up. "I appreciate your honesty. I'm upset the doctor didn't tell us. It sounds like the best thing to do. I wanted to bring him home anyway. Let me talk to the rest of the family."

"Call me or come by and let me know what I can do to help," she said.

I talked to the family and went with the nurse's lead. I asked her to please reschedule a meeting with the hospitalist doctor right away while we waited for the hospice evaluation. It took a few hours before the doctor came in. I walked to the hallway with him.

"Doctor, the discharge nurse tells me Mark probably only has six months to live, and we are delaying the inevitable with a feeding tube. Do you concur?"

"Yes," he said, not keeping eye contact.

"Why didn't you say that to me in the first place?"

He said nothing. His 6' 2" frame towered over me, but I stared right up at him.

He went right into the next thing and asked if I got an appointment with the pain management doctor. Simply, unconscionable! To this day, I have not forgotten the conversation with him in that hallway, not far from Mark's room. He was an asshole at the very moment I needed comfort and a small lifeline to clasp.

The discharge nurse ordered the hospice evaluation, and if the representative came on that day, Mark might get discharged in a few hours or the next day. While my guts turned to water, I attempted to breathe and prepare for the next stage of our husband and wife's journey together. I would help my sweetheart, my greatest love die. The hospice agent showed up. We waited for Mark's evaluation and the consultation on his pain medications. I was in a state of floatation, above water, below water, somewhere else entirely, sharks circling, seagulls screeching. My head numb and tingly, but I had to function. There was no one else who would do this for Mark. I had to do it. I was his angel and he was mine.

While we waited for the hospice care organization's formal approval, I ran through all the list of things to do. I arranged for additional help at home to lift him, which required at least two caregivers, each with a twelve-hour shift. With my brain spinning, I had no idea what to purchase. It began with: A budget to figure out money needs, coordination of

SECTION 3 - HOSPITAL & ASSISTED LIVING

medical care items provided at home by the hospice organization, and move the furniture, clothes, pictures from the shadow box at the assisted living facility. I wanted Mark to see his children and grandchildren on the wall until they came into town.

During this time, while I floundered like a wounded lioness protecting her cubs. Mark's brother Robert, his wife Fran, his sister Pauline and my daughter Ann, were always available while I ran errands, coordinated travel times, made phone calls in preparation for Mark's coming home for his final months. I became his champion, his defender, his rock of Gibraltar who would love him from this life into another.

On that particular day, Mark's brother Robert was with Mark while I went home to shower and clean out Mark's bedroom. Time slipped away quickly, and I hoped the next day didn't come too soon, leaving me ragged and breathless, running from one end of the house to the other. Pauline helped me with at least three trips back and forth to move the clothes, take down a wall of family pictures and empty the shadow entry box. Robert stayed with Mark and waited until I returned to the hospital and didn't leave to have dinner with his wife until someone relieved him. Since it was late, Mark's sister relieved him at the hospital to give me more time, a lifesaver until I went back to Mark at 9:00 p.m.

When I returned, I hugged Mark and his sister. I noticed Mark's food tray still out with untouched soup, and a written note said, "He's waiting to have dinner with his wife."

I picked up the soup and went to the nurse's station. "Can you please heat this for my husband? He hasn't eaten it yet." I thought no one's fault, not enough hours in the day. Not enough hours ever again in a day.

"Sure," the nurse said. I thanked her and went back into the room.

"Honey, I'm sorry no one noticed you hadn't eaten yet. I was busy getting your room ready. You might be able to come home. Would you like that? Would you like to come home?" My eyes were downturned. My voice, a little girl's. I asked him to come home apologetically because I fully expected him to refuse.

"Yes," Mark replied. I couldn't believe it. He understood what I asked him to do.

"I'm giving you the best room with a view of the garden," I said.

SECTION 3 - HOSPITAL & ASSISTED LIVING

The nurse came in with the warmed soup, and I fed it to him. I wanted to cry, and his sister felt terrible, she didn't notice it either. No one at fault; everyone was living on spent energy. I lived on what you called energy but after that; war ripped combat fatigue.

* * *

To cope with Mark's 24/7 care, I pulled hard on the times I helped my Uncle Sal with his meals. Sal, my favorite uncle, was on hospice care at home with ALS. He started having health issues when he approached seventy, but initial tests didn't reveal the diagnosis. Sal never complained during those visits. While he could still talk, we reminisced of the old days with the family and about my mom. I loved those talks.

Mark and I drove two hours to the Bay Area for our periodic visits. I remember how Mark watched Sal's entire transition from lucid and strong to lucid and a near physical vegetable over several months Mark always so kind, joked around with my uncle. It became a regular dare between Mark and Sal, first to phone each other and bet on a game and second to visit Sal and pay up last. Somehow, Uncle Sal always won.

My aunts and I took turns while we trimmed and filed his fingernails. While he still talked, being an engineer, he always said, "Make sure my nails are at a ninety-degree angle." I remember thinking, how tough it is for his out of town kids to visit often. I know they love him. My aunt said she hurt for him, and so did I. I was close to my uncle and got even closer during his illness. Like my parents, he wanted his kids to have the things he didn't have as a child. He was a great, great man, like Mark.

Mark met Sal and my family at our wedding. My uncle loved his engineering work and was a workaholic, but made time to attend our wedding. He had so much in common with Mark. They both enjoyed sports, traveling, fishing, and hunting. Before uncle Sal got sick, I knew someday Mark would enjoy doing things with Sal. Up to that point, he was healthy and never ill. Suddenly taken to the hospital, they discovered heart problems, necessitating bypass surgery. A long inflatable rubber sheet covered his lower limbs to prevent a blood clot in his legs.

SECTION 3 - HOSPITAL & ASSISTED LIVING

Sal, like Mark, a modest man, had never been in the hospital. He dealt with nurses attending to all his private body parts. Discharged from the hospital, Sal continued to see specialists, because he still had a drag in his leg. Unfortunately, after two years and several visits to specialists at Stanford University, he was diagnosed with Lou Gehrig's disease. He worked as long as he could, maybe a year after his diagnosis. Then, afterward, he was cared for at home initially by his retired older sister, then later, with the help of hired in-home caregivers.

My uncle still smiled and even tried to laugh, but it was difficult. I silently said to myself; this is no life for him. Being wheeled in to watch his favorite sports channel or watch a movie. He didn't dress, eat, or drink by himself. His feeding tube hung down from a stainless-steel pole down to his stomach and went everywhere with him. A sight I never wanted to see again.

His only function, his mind, it kept going. He understood everything. To help communicate on some level, my aunt made a board of commands for his needs. He pointed to his wants if he needed to visit the men's room with yes or no responses. He later couldn't talk. He had to be very frustrated, but he never showed it. Eventually, he couldn't even do that, and his hands and feet became stiff and folded inward.

We were told his life with this illness would last two to three years. During those three years, he went from eating, drinking, conversing, to choking on water, then, finally he was on a feeding tube.

Often, I thought I wished I could have said to him, when you get to Heaven, tell my mom and dad I miss and love them. I never said it to him out loud because it sounded so final.

Hospice nurses came in periodically to attend to his needs, as his vital organs were shutting down. Once his feeding tube removed, the nurses said he would have a more peaceful death. I don't remember if it was two or three days after the feeding tube was gone. He finally passed and went to Heaven.

After reflecting on this tragedy, I knew my uncle's death prepared me for Mark's transition from the hospital. No feeding tube became a line I would not cross.

Those words, he would have a more peaceful death without the feeding tube, were embedded in my memory. It was true for my precious Uncle Sal. And now my husband as well.

* * *

I wanted Mark comfortable, without pain, peaceful and with his family for however long we had. We all held him, cared for him, and loved him, while he still breathed the same air with his family and close friends. That envelope of cherished time was closed off to us. We trusted that God held the reopening of his celebration at his will.

SECTION 4 - HOSPICE CARE AT HOME

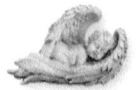

Chapter 24: Hospice Care
[JULY 2012]

The guest bedroom faced our glorious windows. I imagined Mark's gaze following the path of my gaze, his face tilted to the right as he lay in bed. I liked the way the light hit this room, sun slants of pure gold color and warmth, toward the East, protected somewhat from the shade of the trees. I made a mental note the Nandina plants rose a little high above the window sill and needed trimming. The beautiful room was Mark's, and he was to be taken care of and loved and made to feel whole.

Exhausted but in a peaceful place, my cell interrupted my thoughts. It was Robert on the phone.

"Mark will be transported home from the hospital sometime between 5:30 and 6:00 p.m. You have about half an hour to an hour. Are you ready?" He asked with a hint of excitement. He loved his brother and wanted Mark's last months to be comfortable too. It was July 31, 2012, and Mark had been away from home over three months.

"Almost, just a couple more…"

"What?"

"…things to do."

"Okay. Good."

"Umm. Hey, is everything set up with the cable?" I took a deep breath.

"Don't worry. I'll double-check it," voice strong and reassuring.

"Thanks so much. Will you come alongside the transport van?"

"Of course, I'll follow them," he said.

I walked into the hallway toward the entry. The glass-top wrought-iron sofa table was in the way with a small walk-through space between it and the love seat, and a step-down from the entryway. I visualized Mark brought in on the stretcher. Thank God the sofa had button slides at the bottom of the wooden legs, it could easily be pushed on the wood floors to make room. The table a different story, I placed a blanket underneath both sets of legs to drag and pull the blanket on one end.

SECTION 4 - HOSPICE CARE AT HOME

I walked back into the guest bedroom and looked at all the family pictures on the South wall, a perfect view from Mark's extra-long hospital bed. Pauline helped move them from the facility.

Along with the bed, the Hospice organization brought a standing oxygen tank, bed pads, disposable underwear, lotion, and moisture salve for his lips. Fran brought checkered twin sheets for his bed. I pictured Mark on the bed. I took one last survey on top of the dresser, a box of wet wipes, tissues, and lotions. The living room chair and ottoman brought in for caregivers and guests. I did one more peruse in the room. The hospital bed frame had levers and adjusters that moved up and down. I made sure there was enough space on each side for the caregivers to stand and turn him from side to side?

I whispered, "I love you, Mark. I love you."

My heart couldn't take the strain of both having and losing him. I hugged myself hard and then made myself busy.

Quickly I went into the garage and grabbed the clippers to trim the shrubs evenly with the window sill, so Mark could see the flowers and trees he loved. Then I swept the sidewalks, stood, and looked around and thought of the days we worked on the yard together.

Suddenly, I heard engine sounds of gears changing and brakes. I walked through the gate and saw the transport van pulled into the driveway. I secured the gate to stay open and waited inside for Mark. My eyes watered, and tears held back. As the two transport guys held Mark high and carried him into the courtyard, I saw the stress on his crinkled face. His cheeks flushed red, his eyes squinted, and he frowned. This August day scorched anything breathless, and the trip in the van probably bumped all the way. I smiled and welcomed him in.

Would I be a stranger to him? Or would he remember? I'm your loving wife.

I can't remember what the faces of the transport men looked like, except they were tall and strong enough to carry almost two hundred pounds. After they positioned him on the bed, I leaned over, gave him a hug and kiss, and adjusted his sheets and pillows.

"Welcome home, honey, I love you. Want something to drink?"

"Yes," he said.

SECTION 4 - HOSPICE CARE AT HOME

"Do you know where you are?"

"Yes," he said. It was enough for me.

Robert came inside. "Well, you sure know how to make an entrance." He smiled at his brother, and they both laughed. Robert set the tv and took charge of tackling the remote and worked the controls.

The attendants packed up.

"Can we get you some water before you leave?" Robert asked them.

The attendants shook their heads and smiled. "No, thanks," the bigger one said. "We have water in the van. Can we help you move anything?" My thoughts: I sure could have used your help before.

I got a small dampened towel and placed it on Mark's face to cool him. In the background, I heard the rumble of the transport van leave and drift away. I looked at Mark with a sigh of relief, and he looked back at me silently with his green eyes, and I thought his eyes said, I'm happy I'm home. Then I heard the pleasant sound of soft music off of the cable music station.

"Hey Robert, thanks so much for the nice sound! The timing was perfect," I said.

"You bet!" He said with a large smile.

Then I mixed Mark's special thick water-nutrition-goop and spoon-fed him. It was hard doing that. Mark wasn't my child. He was my husband.

Later that day and the following days, I received phone calls from the hospice team of angels. No stones unturned, first the nurse called to set up the initial visit.

The hospice social worker called to set an appointment for the preparations on the next phase of Mark's journey to Heaven. She arrived, and I invited her in. We sat in the living room and she handed me a fold-out brochure, the last thing I wanted - more to read.

"These are a few things to decide. I'll read the questions outlined, but you don't need to answer anything now, I know this is overwhelming. Here they are: Have you made future funeral arrangements? Has a pastor been selected? Are all your legal papers in order? Can we help you with personal respite time?" While she spoke, I couldn't give her complete eye contact. I looked back and forth at her, then to all our family photos on the hutch. I didn't want to talk. My hands gripped tightly.

SECTION 4 - HOSPICE CARE AT HOME

"I appreciate you taking this time to help us. I'll make sure to go over this with my family. Right now, it doesn't seem real. I can't pull my thoughts together to make any sense of this." I said. It felt the conversation was about someone else.

I still had nagging thoughts embedded in my head of the last week before Mark came home from the hospital on hospice care. The doctor's loud words, the way he spoke to me in the hallway about his suggestions for Mark to go on a feeding tube. And when I walked back into Mark's room, he said he didn't want a bird feeder. I didn't want that either. I was stunned and shocked.

What I didn't tell the social worker was that my husband was very private, and I had to be present most when he's being changed, or he got combative with the caregivers, as he had done in the hospital.

"About the support, I do have my family, my daughter, his brother, his wife, and his sister. So, you see, I do have lots of support. Thank you, though." I said after a long hesitation.

Shortly after that, the hospice doctor called to set an appointment for the next day to evaluate Mark. An Asian female doctor arrived. After the introductions, I asked her inside, and we sat at the dining room table. She had a very soft and sensitive sounding voice and looked like a friend coming to visit in casual pants and a white blouse. She declined my offer of something to drink and pulled a notebook from her briefcase.

Her first question, "When did you start noticing problems?"

"About six years ago," I swallowed and said.

"What kinds of things did you notice him do differently?" She looked at me with sympathetic eyes.

I hesitated to gather my thoughts, then replied. "Mark's been repeating things. His short-term memory is bad. His physical body is bad with chronic back and neck pain. He walks with a gaited-limp in his legs. He sees invisible people. He had bad allergies and asthma before."

"Does he remember you?" she asked.

"Yes, but within the past four months, his grandchildren came to visit, and I don't know if he remembered them all," I said.

"How many children are there?" She flipped her notebook to another page.

"He has two daughters, and I have one daughter," I said while she wrote things down on her notes.

"I'd like to evaluate Mark first, and then I'll circle back to you."

I nodded, by deliberately moving my head up and down. I got up and asked her to follow me, then walked her into his room.

"Mark, this is the doctor. She needs to ask you a few questions. I'll leave you alone for a few minutes." I walked back into the living room and sat on the sofa.

I didn't hear any words while I waited, but I heard the door open after a few minutes and heard her footsteps in the hallway. I asked her to the dining room table for more privacy and again asked if she wanted anything to drink, but she declined. She followed, and we sat at the table.

"Based on my evaluation, his mobility problems might indicate Mark has a Lewy Body Dementia. That disease afflicts the physical body faster than Alzheimer's Dementia."

I steeled myself for more pain and terror. "Doctor, that makes sense to me, but the UCSF Alzheimer's center concluded he had Alzheimer's Dementia. We'll know for sure after he passes. We signed papers to donate his brain for research and science. In turn, we're supposed to get a full report of the autopsy, showing the cause of death. What you're saying makes a lot of sense, though." I said, trying not to collapse under the table. I learned of this disease in workshops I attended, and it made sense. Mark continued to know me, but his body had many physical problems with a dragging gait, and his neck and back aching. It struck me, nothing was certain, as my heart pounded. I paused and then swallowed.

"Sure, sure," she said. "When I asked Mark how old he was and how many children he has, he said, "I'm thirty-five, and I have three children.""

"Doctor, Mark is seventy." Heartburn roared inside my chest. I took the plunge. "How much time do we have with him?"

"Six days to six months. It's hard to give you more than that," she replied with slight hesitation.

Six days to six months, hard to give me more than that. After I heard those words, I was motionless, my head was full, yet light and numb, in moments of absorption, like being sucked away in a vacuum and incapable of breathing and in no uncertain terms, dying myself.

SECTION 4 - HOSPICE CARE AT HOME

The days were full, and my heart struggled for strength, all the while steeling myself for what was to come with Mark. If anyone thinks there is some 'magical' balanced point of acceptance, good luck with that. As within the hospital, I continued to help the caregivers at changing or turning times. It was such a relief to know they sat with Mark 24/7 to keep him company and let me know if Mark needed anything while I was out of the room doing other things. People imagine when home with your loved one, somehow allows you time to rest or sit on the couch and watch television, pay your bills, or accomplish any number of projects from home. And often that can be true. But when you're in love for the long run, when your guts are ripped out your ribcage, and then you realize you're a ghost in the wind, tethered to the ground in stages or floating far above the room. And no matter what was going on, you must function, function, function. It was grueling, spirit robbing and more than I could bear. As well as Mark's 'new normal,' my 'new normal' was, I became someone else who I didn't recognize. Scrawny, ashen, pale, wounded to my core, unearthed. Wishing with all of my heart Mark and I would be together forever.

I had to let him go. Alone.

The hospice nurse arrived with her bundle of pain medications. She was young, heavyset, and full of knowledge, shared all the instructions on how to administer to Mark. She also left a booklet to read, about the stages of further deterioration with pain Mark would experience. I was to watch for his signs, symptoms, and body language, which aided me in making sure the cocktail of medications was enough, or if we had to increase this or that. He continued with his regular asthma and reflux meds, but after a few days, I wondered if he should continue them with the pain management meds. He took a total of ten different meds for pain, nausea, congestion, itching, and shortness of breath. A real awakening to realize his pain management was dependent on the watchful eye of the caregivers and me. I had no idea hospice at home was such a huge responsibility, and I was completely swallowed by it. I had assistance from the hospice nurse on call any time. The hospice nurses visited our home once or twice in the beginning and came more frequently when closer to Mark's passing. Left up to me to lead in pain management was another that said, 'I was there to take away his pain' while my pain climbed through the heavens. There was no cure, no magic pill or magic treatment that would make him better. I'd used up any bargaining with God. All I could do at this stage was get down on my knees and pray for courage.

Fortunately, I hired two caregivers from the independent assisted living organization; one started the first evening at 9:00 p.m. She was a heavyset, middle-aged African American woman with a large smile named Bobbie. I welcomed her and asked her to have a seat. I explained Mark's health condition and how I wanted her to spend time talking to him and attending to his needs while I was not in his room. I wanted her to make sure he was always comfortable, clean and his underwear was changed. Often, the nurse's aide and the caregiver referred to the underwear as diapers, and I didn't like Mark heard it, so I asked them to refer to as underwear.

"Mark's tall body slides down the bed and needs adjusting sometimes, and his feet come close to the foot of the bed. So, please watch him. He's also very private, so let me know when you need me. That way, I can be present to help calm him down, while you change and clean him," I explained.

"Sure will, Miss Jean," Bobbie said.

I showed her the extra bedroom for her breaks, the bathroom, and the kitchen. Then I took her into the bedroom and introduced her to Mark. Mark seemed to like her, and he smiled and said hello. After I left the room, I began to read the hospice booklet provided. In the background, I heard Mark talking to Bobbie, and I was relieved. He sprouted the root of new energy; he was home. I went into his room later, holding a glass of wine to say goodnight with a kiss.

"Can I have some wine?" he said.

He wanted to partake in our occasional evening ritual of wine and appetizers. I was overwhelmed with emotion and all the responsibility. I wanted to give him that wine but knew I shouldn't. Instead, I offered him a frozen smoothie. I left the room and returned with the smoothie and fed it to him in small bites with a spoon.

"This is better. Doesn't that taste great?" I said, and he nodded yes.

It was up to me to administer his medications. I organized a way to document his ten medications, when he took them, how much to give him, and suddenly I wondered if he needed to continue his regular medications? I called the hospice doctor and asked if it was necessary. She said no, only hospice pain management prescriptions were needed.

My instruction booklet indicated he wasn't capable of letting me know if he was hurting at some point. His actions showed if he needed more or not. If he looked distressed or waved his hands, that was my sign, his dosage was not enough, and I called for an increase from the doctor. I kept an eye on his bladder and bowel movements.

The next day a new caregiver arrived, this time a younger, almost shy, Hispanic woman. I went through the same drill with her. I attended Mark to make sure he had everything needed. I wasn't sure how he took to different caregivers at different shifts, but if they were friendly, attentive, and conscientious, I felt it worked well. Until one day, when it didn't work at all.

The tobacco-smelling caregiver came. A middle-aged, hyperactive male, though a sensitive guy, reeked of cigarettes. The same day, the pointed acrylic nail caregiver with a stink-fest of flowery cologne arrived. It didn't work with a conflicting set of bad odors. I wasn't exposing Mark to the awful gray cloud attack of the ashtray smelling caregiver, nor allow the pointed acrylic nail caregiver to turn Mark with her spiked claws. I gently advised the agency to let both of them go immediately.

"No problem, we'll send someone else." The owner apologized for the pointed acrylic nail caregiver, who filled in for someone. After that, I realized specific orders for their services were necessary and they would accommodate.

I was thankful for the continued support and thoughtfulness by Ann, Robert, Fran, and Pauline during all the hospital visits, Ann religiously was at my side, while Robert and Pauline visited daily and kept conversations light. They were my support team, and I could count on them for anything. In the three hospital visits, while I stayed with Mark, Fran brought me a vanilla latte and oatmeal every morning She was thoughtful and knew I skipped meals during that time.

After Mark came home on hospice, Fran thought of everything, even getting an electric wet one warmer. It kept the wet ones warm, before touching Mark's body to clean him. We wanted him comfortable and kept

SECTION 4 - HOSPICE CARE AT HOME

him dressed in his regular button-down shirts. We slit his shirts in the back; so they could be removed with ease. Pauline lost her husband from cancer. She was always helpful, giving insightful advice and knew just what to say.

Mark's daughters and their families arrived. They arranged to stay with his brother during the next few weeks. They brought the grandchildren every day to see Mark, and he could see and hear their energetic voices and laughter while they moved around his bed.

They played Mark's favorite music from Neil Diamond and Tony Bennett, songs their dad played during their childhood days. They sang to him and showered him with the love he knew was always there. Mark had a renewed sense of awareness during the first week. He heard the sounds he wished he could have heard more every day, but couldn't because of the logistics of his kids five hours away.

He finally saw his latest grandchildren, the twins, who were born three months before. Their mother, Jill, held them each individually and leaned them over, one at a time to her dad, as he kissed each of them. It was a cloud of tears from everyone in the room. I wondered how much could be embedded in their infant souls of his instant love for his family before he went to the next stage of his life.

Then, of all times, the air conditioning fan blew out hot air. I stood outside in the heat, waiting for a report of what was needed when the repairman said I needed a new main electrical breaker. It was a Saturday and almost impossible to get an electrician to work on the weekend.

"Ma'am, because there's a wire seal over it, it requires city approval before anyone can work on it," he said.

"Oh no! I'll call their emergency line," I called the City and stated our situation, but the representative sounded cavalier.

"I'm sorry ma'am, we can't get anyone over there until Monday."

"If you don't get someone over here right now during our emergency, I'll break the seal myself. My husband can't be in a 100-plus degree heat on hospice care!" With sweat dripping off my forehead, flushed and angry, I yelled. The fatigue overtook me. I completely lost it.

"Okay, ma'am, I'll get someone right over there," Absolutely you shit brick asshole.

SECTION 4 - HOSPICE CARE AT HOME

Our usual electrician, who didn't work on Saturdays, came with a new breaker after receiving my desperate phone call and replaced the main breaker. I went back into the house while the company kept Mark occupied, and I walked into the kitchen. Fran was in the kitchen, filling the water canister when I approached her and went to pieces. I shook and wept, the most I cried from the time of Mark's diagnosis. I finally let go and released it. Fran walked to me and hugged me as I wept, wept, and shook almost to the point of fainting. All this, while close friends in the living room sat and allowed me privacy in the kitchen to mourn this horrible nightmare. As the days went by, it was as though I was outside of my body, only to observe it going through the motions, not aware of my direction and the timing of it all. After a few minutes, Fran offered me a glass of water.

"Why don't you go take a shower? Maybe it'll help you," she said.

"Yes, I think I will, before the kids come back," I panted and stumbled out of the kitchen.

It wasn't long before all of Mark's nieces, nephews and more friends came to visit. One friend even sang a song, "Knowing You," to Mark. I didn't know he had such a good voice. The same friend honored when I asked him to shave Mark.

It was a good day for Mark. He said a few words and looked at me with love.

"I want somebody someday to look at me the way Uncle Mark looks at you!" one of his nieces said. I felt lucky that God chose Mark for me, even if it was for a short fifteen years.

His skin looked better, full of color and light than it had in weeks. He was happy and comfortable that first week. He had eaten some mashed potatoes and creamed chicken soup for the first six days. On the 7th day, he lost his appetite. He only wanted thick liquids, mostly frozen smoothies.

I made a chart to track the medication times and meals eaten, to keep everyone aware of Mark's status.

Mark ended up with 10 different caregivers, less the two dismissed for tobacco and sharp acrylic nails. There were usually two per day, each with a 12-hour swift. Towards the end, two caregivers in the morning and the evenings helped turn Mark's body. We were lucky to have caregivers well suited for this job. They were very conscientious, thoughtful, and empathetic. They offered to do housework or anything we needed while they were not attending to Mark.

Days went by, and Mark talked less and less. Telepathic messages from me to him and from him to me were the strongest medication I could give him. He was close to death. My man was dying. We tried to keep him pain-free, but at the same time, we were navigating his journey to the other side. He would need to leave this world to enter the next one. At times, I had extreme pressure in my chest, but it was our duty. He was my duty and my love. I would not let him down.

SECTION 4 - HOSPICE CARE AT HOME

SECTION 4 - HOSPICE CARE AT HOME

Chapter 25: Decisions
[AUGUST 2012]

Mark's younger daughter, Tammy, studied nursing. She said if his urine was amber-colored, it indicated he was closer to passing. The first week of August 2012 went by. Mark had not eaten much and no bowel movement since he came home.

"Has he had a bowel movement?" The nurse asked.

"No," I said.

"We might want to give him a suppository."

"Why do we need to put him through that?" Tammy said.

"I agree," I said. We never gave it to him. At that point, it seemed like placing a grain of sand into the white waters of a moving river.

* * *

There were many things to plan concurrently, and most of them had to do with Mark's passing. Dread filled me. I already buried my parents, which prepared me to coordinate Mark's service and took me to a spiritual place where I whispered and pleaded for God's certain grace. The topics involving Mark's service were endless and taxing. Pain entered my heart with spider legs, injected venom, burrowed into my flesh.

The entire family gathered one day and selected a family pastor who knew Mark's children. I asked his daughters to assemble a video with music and pictures. Ann and Robert helped me look for available churches for the service, just in case the church we married in was not available.

Again, I felt I was dying too.

How could I bury the man I loved in the same church that forever bound us in love?

Suggestions kept coming. Fran mentioned a catered family dinner at a restaurant. A good idea, but I wanted an outdoor dinner, where green was a life that Mark loved. I selected the centerpiece flowers, but mostly with greenery like the mountains.

SECTION 4 - HOSPICE CARE AT HOME

Since our church was not available, we looked at three available churches. The last one gave me a message. We waited outside of the church; I heard the sound of a flock of ducks or geese flying over the church, it was very clear to Ann and me, Mark said, 'Pick this church.' His extensive collection of duck decoys displayed in our home was always a joke when my young grandchildren visited. They always said, "Grandma Jean, does Mark like ducks?"

"There's our sign. Mark wants this church," I said while I looked at Ann.

"It sure is." Ann shook her head up and down.

As soon as Robert arrived, we went into the church office. Greeted by a friendly young woman, perfect for the job, she wondered how many we estimated would attend, and was it breakfast or lunch? She offered available times and said the meal would be served and cleaned by their staff. After the celebration of life, a luncheon followed the church service next door in the assembly hall. It sounded perfect; all I needed was to designate someone in the family to move flowers home from the service. We walked into the small chapel with lots of windows, lightly filtered inside as a symbol from God, and it accommodated 400 people. It was perfect.

* * *

The shifts of caregivers changed every three days. I was thankful for the caregiver during the evenings; she was perfect. Aria was a young woman with soulful eyes, a sweet demeanor, a confident voice, and blessed with caring hands. I had a strong connection to her and was happy that God placed her with us.

It was more and more challenging when I tried to figure out if I should increase Mark's dosage. With his eyebrows furrowing or when he raised his hand, he gave us signs, so I called the nurse to get confirmation to increase the dosage. Mark couldn't talk, and I wanted him to pass without pain. I heard my internal, harsh nagging voice; you're killing him with the pain management. Even though I knew it was to help, for him to die less painfully.

SECTION 4 - HOSPICE CARE AT HOME

"Don't you think we should be giving him more?" his daughter Tammy expressed that particular day.

In frustration, I said, "Then why don't you call the hospice nurse and ask her?" Tammy did, and the dosage increased.

Without it said, the signs were apparent. The time was near. Mark hadn't spoken much in at least five days.

I had my schedule set every night. I went to bed around 10:00, slept for a few hours, then went into Mark's room, every three hours, unless the caregiver came sooner than instructed. I told the caregiver to let me know if she needed help, or if his breathing sounded different. Mark no longer swallowed and got doses of pain medication every three hours. It was mixed with water and put into small syringes, dropped under his tongue. It permeated his membranes faster to relieve his pain. Death is a painful process.

It was always tricky measuring the medication, making sure it was the right consistency and dosage, squeezing the dropper into his mouth. I always second-guessed myself with the thoughts of: Did I get it right? Will it relieve him? Is it burning his mouth?

* * *

I went through a process when Ann had mono as a teenager. I gave her injections and made sure no bubbles were in the syringe. I always tapped the needle until finally, Ann shouted, "Mom, just give it to me!" I wasn't good with shots or anything related to medications. It all came from a place as a toddler in line with my parents, lied to about a shot I was told I didn't need. I ran away quickly but was retrieved and given the ugly, painful shot. I never got over it and certainly didn't want to anoint anyone else with the pain. My parents never meant harm, but as a child, it stayed present and screamed out at inopportune times. Plus, I was a klutz with needles. Honestly, I sucked at being his nurse.

* * *

SECTION 4 - HOSPICE CARE AT HOME

I couldn't get over giving my soul mate, the love of my life, the man that made me so happy, shots and syringes that meant deception, pain, and death. I wanted to run again and I couldn't.

At the end of the day shift, the caregiver and I turned Mark's body to the other side. Aria arrived for her evening shift, greeted Mark and touched his hands. This woman was in the right profession. She had perfect listening skills, empathy, and love to handle this delicate situation of a women's husband passing on to Heaven. This poor young Aria, who had young children, was here to help me take care of Mark.

I left to wash my hands. When I returned, Aria sat on the floor, the way she did on previous nights, leaning on the chest of drawers with a tablet of paper on her lap. I sat next to her on the floor, and we talked. I heard her life story about her family and their dreams. I shared stories about our short, married life before Mark got diagnosed.

"I can't believe you were only married six short years before his diagnosis," she said.

"Yes, Aria. We had the best six years. We had fun traveling. We especially liked the simple, inexpensive hiking trips in the mountains. Try to keep your life simple. Most of all, our love and respect for one another has sustained and deepened throughout this time in our lives. Let me tell you about our last trip to Montana."

* * *

Funny to be so happy in the glorious mountains of Montana in 2005 and so nervous about Mark.

My outdoor athletic husband forgot things. He made light of it. I could not. Nervous, I decided it was stress from other family issues.

I thought a trip would help. Mark was just too tired.

Mark excelled on adventure trips, hunted deer and fished in oceans and lakes. I suggested a Montana or Wyoming vacation. I wanted an easy-going trip, no fancy clothes, and the same pair of jeans we would wear into the mud. I researched the area for historical facts, found where Lewis and Clark navigated and mapped a path through the continental divide.

SECTION 4 - HOSPICE CARE AT HOME

We invited our good friends, Sonny and Betty, to join us. A glimpse of this couple was summed up in Betty's car license plate, "CRZYLDY."

I'd marked stars on a map for our route. Internet showed postcard scenes with the wide-open spaces of the Big Sky land, with wildflowers of pink, yellow and purple, green pastures, mountains, elk, bison, and lots of big sunny skies.

Mark reserved a boat from the River Rat expedition in Craig, Montana equipped with oars, floatation vests, and fishing poles.

Near the sandy and rocky shore of the river, we waited on a grassy shoreline. Surprised and greeted by a thinly framed, grandfatherly man with bright, inquisitive, eyes who wore a weather-stained cowboy hat, boots, and overalls. He was a retired engineer. He looked old to run rivers.

Backing his truck up to the water, he unloaded the boat.

Mark jokingly barked orders, "Girls will paddle! Men will fish!"

"Who called you captain?" Betty said as she snickered.

No one knew weather conditions, but who cared. We soon found out what we were made of, and who'd catch the first fish. Fastened in our yellow life jackets, the girls jumped in first. Nodding, I dug into the oar, followed the movement of my gloved hands.

Such a wide river, we went around an island to get on the right side. We worked hard to fight the ferocious current and the commanding wind that pummeled against us. Casts flew in every direction. The fishing lines flew back in the opposite direction.

We maneuvered to the river edge. My body felt bludgeoned. Back muscles in spasm, palms locking up.

We paddled with all we had to the other side. Not unhappy to cut our excursion short, we looked forward to the help of the River Rat, who was waiting. Sweaty, windburned, and still sassy, we piled into his truck.

Thankful, we offered to buy the River Rat a drink and asked about the closest bar. All equipment stored, we walked to our cars up the dirt path. We noticed new buildings to the left and an older set on the right. We chose the neighborhood barn for the local spirit.

Greeted by a white-haired woman bartender at the U-shaped bar as well as characters out of a western comedy with boots and spurs and serious poker faces, we were thrilled to the bone.

SECTION 4 - HOSPICE CARE AT HOME

"Let the fun begin!" Mark announced.

It did. Mark was a natural in this rural cowboy environment.

The local farmer with jean overalls, boots, and a cowboy hat came to sell his produce. He lay the box on the counter with leafy greens that hung off the sides. River Rat bought eggs, potatoes, onions, peppers. He looked at us. I thought he must be expecting some company, that's a lot for one person.

"Why don't you folks have dinner at my place? Spend the night. Don't drive." Presumed, we'd accept.

"We don't have far to go. Thanks anyway," Mark politely said.

Nice thought, but we each looked at each other. It was not happening. The curious trust the River Rat offered was a little too strange. Sadly, we didn't accept the invitation.

* * *

Driving west to reach the South end of Flathead Lake near Big Fork, the last leg of the trip, elation, and fatigue made us giddy with camping songs.

Into a little village with two blocks of shops, we looked at Indian turquoise jewelry, and shopkeepers directed us to have dinner later at the only local pizzeria/bar on the Southeast side of the four corners.

I looked toward my husband. He seemed fine. Was he?

Strangers in this Big Sky territory, and we met a local developer in a bar in Kalispell, Montana. Mark accepted his open-door invitation. We lived boldly with the locals, and the developer drove us to his house.

We walked into the two-story house of the developer, a John Wayne look-a-like, to an obvious game room with television, ping pong table, and sleeping quarters upstairs. All wide-eyed, we saw the massive moose heads, a mountain lion on a pedestal on the wall, and listened to the developer's big stories.

Two hours later, ready for our return trip, he refused to drive us. "Just take my car. Leave the keys under the mat." We looked at each other in shock. He handed Mark the keys. After hugs and handshakes, we walked some minutes through pitch blackness. We held hands and found our way to the car. Mark, like a true navigator, led us back to the bar.

No longer strangers, we realized there was trust among us in the "Big Sky" with the people in Flathead Lake. Like most things, it took time to build that confidence with the Montanans on that last leg of the trip.

* * *

A few months after this breathtaking journey, Mark was diagnosed with Early Onset Alzheimer's. I needed the memories of our wilderness trip to Montana and the outright kindness shown to us, by strangers, to strengthen me while my sweet, precious husband lost his memories of our lives together. And it did. As we paddled down the river, fighting to hold on, visions of the Montana sky never left me. Gratitude-gratitude. My love for Mark was as strong as the fiercest river current in Montana.

SECTION 4 - HOSPICE CARE AT HOME

SECTION 4 - HOSPICE CARE AT HOME

Chapter 26: Release
[AUGUST 2012]

I went to bed after all the storytelling with Aria. My bond with Aria gave me a sense of comfort, ease, and trust. I knew Mark heard me talk of such pride about our relationship, even though he couldn't speak, he knew I was near. I lay in bed and knew I had to walk my love through the transition to a better place. At the same time, I thought, How can I? I wanted to escape with him and couldn't bear the thought of being left alone without him. He understood me and loved me for me. I wondered, will God allow him to be with me, in the quiet or silence perhaps, to help guide me through my transition without him? After my mom passed, I received a message in a dream. I heard her words as if she was in my room, 'That's okay, Jean. Everything is going to be all right.' I could only hope for his message or messages.

I looked at him at night, still as stone, he didn't move, but his chest rose up and down in slow rhythm, barely breathing. I hoped he smelled me and sensed I was there. Even though he was leaving, in my heart, I knew he would go to Heaven. I had conflicting thoughts of letting him go, he had been here only two weeks in August 2012, but I had to release him from the pain he endured. I couldn't bring myself to talk to him.

The book from the hospice organization said he needed to know I released him. I wondered, "Have his kids talked to him, his brother, his sister, and his friends? We were alone, but not the right time. I was in constant thought of all the things I wanted to say to him.

He often talked to me poetically and was always such a wordsmith. This poem he wrote to me:

"I bestowed my frostbitten soul
on you only I know
On you, my thoughts rivet
On you, I grow
The Spring is complete now
Thanks, I give freely"

I often told him he had such flair and sounded European. He inspired me and gave me a sense of pride as a friend and husband. He loved me with all of his heart and couldn't have asked for a better mate than God gave me in our short life. He gave me more than I ever expected.

I walked in and out many times, to touch him gently, kiss his cheek, stroke, and pat his hair back. Sometimes, "I love you." Then on the day I released him, I asked to be alone with him.

"Honey, you know how much I love you. You mean everything to me. You have done everything right and perfect. I couldn't have asked for a better husband and best friend. I know how much pain you have endured. I know I must give you up to God. I don't want you to suffer anymore." Another touch and kiss and I left the room. I walked out with a stillness in my whole body. Numb, yet, wondered if he heard what he needed from the rest of the family and me.

As he lay there on the hospital bed, still and silent, sometimes rotated his right side, with pillows behind his back to hold him up, and sometimes on his left. If on his back, his body slid down with his feet touching the foot of the bed. It took two to three people to pull him back up to the head of the bed. My favorite guy was held up on his side while the bedsheets and pads were changed, rolling him from side to side. With three people lifting, his weight in this state felt like twice the weight.

There were many silent days of no communication. Tammy and Jill had been here for two weeks and visited every day. I had given them alone time to speak with their dad. My Ann spent many nights with me, and she was here this night. I could always count on her. Even though she endured my loud snores, she was faithful. I accidentally called her 'Fanny,' the nickname I'd used when she was young because her fanny was so adorable. She hated it.

"Mom," she said with us cuddling. "You know I hate that name."

"I know, it slipped out," I said.

Mark's children were kind and attentive. It was hard for all of us. "Would you like me to spend the night and help you?" Tammy asked. Like all of us, she had tired lines on her face.

"Yes, I would love that," I replied.

SECTION 4 - HOSPICE CARE AT HOME

We each did a three-hour shift to give Mark his pain medications, then alternated. It was early on Saturday morning, at about 2:55 a.m., right before my turn, when I heard a tap on my bedroom door. Aria said, "He sounds very different." I jumped out of bed quickly and went in. Ann followed me. The death rattle sounds of loud hard bubbly choking breaths approached. Mark took what sounded like his last breaths.

"Go get Tammy," I said to Aria. Tammy ran from her bedroom immediately. Tears rolled down our faces, Tammy and I put our hands on our Mark, and we each told him we loved him, and that he was doing everything right. I leaned over to touch his face, his shoulders, and softly kissed his cheek. Tammy leaned over, kissed her dad, and wept.

We witnessed the transition from enduring days of physical movements of pain to death rattle choking; to utter stillness with no breath, and calm release of the transition to Heaven.

Did he hold out, to continue being with his loved ones on earth, or did he finally find his mom, as he once yelled out to me? "I can't find my mom!"

I responded. "Your mom is in Heaven praying for you. You'll find her."

Was he finally at peace, found his mom, or God waiting for him? Emotional devastation and contradiction for those of us left behind by our loved one going to a better place, without pain, but painful for us without Mark.

Four months from the time of his first hospital visit, he endured pain, separation, and confusion. In total, in and out of the hospital four times, taken from our home to the assisted living and back home on hospice for eighteen days. He deteriorated, unable to communicate those last few days. He hallucinated for at least a year, seeing people, his mom, lost friends, inside the transparent spirit world. I wondered: Were there telepathic messages from those who lived on the other side, to Mark? Were they calling him Home? His spirit transitioned.

I informed the family Mark passed and called the hospice nurse. She came to report the time of death, Saturday, August 18, 2012, at approximately 3:15 a.m. Mark's spirit floated from our house. My fingers trembled, and my eyes watered. I made several phone calls, alerting the funeral home for

SECTION 4 - HOSPICE CARE AT HOME

their verification of his passing. Over and over, I repeated these words. "My husband passed away. My husband passed away."

"This is Mark's wife. My husband just passed away." I said on what seemed like call number twelve.

The nurse tried for my sake. "I'm so sorry. You know he's no longer in pain."

"I know."

"He's in a better place."

"I believe that too."

The family arrived later, and we waited for the funeral representatives. It was again a time of floatation, a stillness in the air. I went through the motions, not understanding how to deal. I walked into the kitchen and back into the bedroom. I had to move, and I became what I wasn't able to control, a pacing animal, a wounded tigress with an arrow in her heart.

Jill arrived first and was more emotional. Her three kids would never know their Grandpa, the dad they admired and loved. It was up to Jill and Tammy to keep his memory alive in their eyes, as a strong and fun-loving Grandpa. She could tease them, perhaps as he teased her and her sister, Tammy.

Robert, Pauline and Fran arrived, then went to Mark, and touched and kissed his face. They comforted Jill, Tammy, Ann and me with hugs and kisses.

I left the room and went to the kitchen. I wanted to be alone. I loved all the support, but at times, I couldn't breathe. I imagined him sitting in his chair and reading his morning newspaper, while he ate his bowl of cereal, as I looked at him with pride. The cozy nook, I sat across from Mark for a few minutes, I was in a cocoon of comfort and safety amidst his spirit.

Pounding on the front door startled us. The funeral representatives and hearse arrived and wheeled in their stretcher to take Mark to the funeral home. They began to wrap and cover him over his underwear and T-shirt.

"Please wait," I said. I stepped in and changed Mark in a clean shirt and long pajama bottoms and covered Mark before they took him. I held him a little longer.

SECTION 4 - HOSPICE CARE AT HOME

I wanted to keep his dignity intact even to the last minute, just once more for my Mark.

At 6:30 a.m., just after daybreak with a slight mist in the air, the family followed in procession. Hand in hand, we gave Mark our love, as the funeral aides wheeled his body to the hearse. Tears rolled down our stoic faces. After 18 days at home, Mark was released with no more pain, and onto Heaven.

Everyone went back inside and offered to help, but I accepted the caregiver, Aria's offer to stay and help. I told everyone thanks, but to go home and shower, I would see them later. We all needed a break.

"Jean, why don't you go take a shower. Let me know what hospice needs for pick up, or if there's anything you need?" Aria asked.

"Thank you so much. I'm glad you're here." I held her hands. Aria was my angel helper, on the way to great things in her own life, but not too hasty to leave and go home.

Aria stayed until 7:30 a.m. While I showered, she organized the items for the hospice organization to pick up. It was a blessing to have her those last few days, especially that morning.

When Aria left, I felt an emptiness. I walked into Mark's bedroom and said a prayer. I released him spiritually, but energy still tugged at my heart.

I sat down and tried long inhales and exhales to help organize my thoughts for the obituary, church service, friends luncheon, caterer for the family dinner, menu, flowers, and what to wear. Overwhelmed, with a week to organize and plan the celebration of Mark's life, I called Fran.

"Fran, it would make me happy if you could write Mark's obituary. Would you?"

"I would be honored to do it," she replied.

His daughters assembled the music video and photographs. They listened to different CDs of music and paired the music to the pictures. I hired the caterer for the family dinner.

At the flower shop, ordering flowers, I saw Mark's ex-sister-law, an identical twin, ordering flowers for Mark's service.

"I'm so sorry for your loss. We loved Mark, and wanted to keep in touch, but didn't want to cause him problems. We won't be attending the

SECTION 4 - HOSPICE CARE AT HOME

service, so my sister won't cause a scene. If you know what I mean," she said. She was estranged from his ex-wife.

"I understand," I answered on rote. I heard stories over the years of their battles, but I was too depressed and miserable to say much more or try to boost the twin sister's spirits. Mine vacant.

* * *

At the service, Tammy asked, "How are you so strong today?" Inside I was a mess, I tried to hold it together but continuously took deep breaths to calm myself. Strength, rarely what it looks like in the movies, but more like a cold bitch. And on this day, I carried her, this heavy, invisible burden in my quivering arms, and praised for it. I don't know why.

The church hosted a luncheon after the service. I wanted the family dinner outdoors. I called all the restaurants with patios, but no availability. I asked our friends, (Montana trip friends) Betty and Sonny, if the dinner could be catered in their backyard. Many parties had been hosted in their beautifully landscaped yard. They were happy to do it.

The caterer handled it all. They brought lights and speakers for the music, which lined the trees and centerpieces for all the tables. The menu for the family dinner was Mark's favorite salmon for the main course, a variety of salads, and his weakness of chocolate desserts.

* * *

I felt Mark was with us in spirit and would have loved that we celebrated his life in the backyard, where he enjoyed many fun times. At the dinner, several family members told stories about Mark, and one of his daughters asked me to speak, but I declined. I wasn't capable of telling any funny or loving stories about my Mark, not just yet. I wanted to be invisible. I medicated myself to a calm, almost stoic state, with many drinks to get through the night. I felt displaced, lonely and out of wits. How could they expect me to tell a story? I felt like screaming, "I want to be with Mark!" I was alone. Alone even though everyone was around me. Hard to explain unless you've been through it yourself.

SECTION 4 - HOSPICE CARE AT HOME

I went through the complex experience of love and sadness, watching loved ones go in different ways, from my mom's accidental death to my father's sudden fatal stroke, and Mark's illness with all the complications.

SECTION 4 - HOSPICE CARE AT HOME

SECTION 5 - AFTER

Chapter 27: Division
[AUGUST 2012]

Mark planned his estate to prevent complications, but emotions and grieving change things that once made sense.

Mark's kids stayed with Robert and Fran. The day after the family dinner, I took leftover food to their house. Tammy walked me to the door. "Can we come over to get the things from my dad's safe and a few things, like the duck decoys?" she asked.

"Sure," I replied. It was the day after, and while my family and friends stayed with me. I didn't mean sure. I thought, what the hell? I didn't mind; they wanted keepsakes, but the timing was difficult. I didn't have a chance to get my grip after the services.

I answered the door. Mark's girls came with their uncle, Robert. The first place they wanted to go was to Mark's safe. I escorted them out to the garage. I watched Robert turn the combination to open the safe. I thought about how Mark wanted to open the safe every day last year. I worried about the guns. The safe had hunting rifles, rolled up coins, his previous wedding band, and a gold nugget ring. They looked surprised and disappointed.

"Your dad gave your aunt and me each a bullion," Robert said. His daughters looked stunned. They surveyed up and around the garage at packed boxes. I never knew, until that morning, Mark previously gave his brother and sister each a silver bullion. His prerogative to give what he wanted, I didn't need to explain anything, but I was uncomfortable.

"Those boxes are Christmas ornaments and my dad's boxes after he passed away. My brother and I need to go through them together," I said. When Mark gave me the combination to the safe, I typed an inventory and made sure Robert got a copy of it. We walked back inside the house. My first awful thought, they think I robbed his safe before they got here.

"I'd like to get a couple of my dad's shirts to make a blanket out of them. Is it okay, Jean?" Tammy said.

SECTION 5 - AFTER

"Sure, go ahead," I said. I was hurt and torn inside, the girls couldn't wait.

"Jill, want any?" Tammy asked.

While they searched, my aunt Terry, my girlfriend, and I sat on the sofa with raised eyebrows. I was silent, while my insides turned inside out. It was their dad, but why couldn't they wait? I thought, do they think I would run off with things meant for them, that I was dishonest? Then, Tammy walked into Mark's office, took a paperweight, and walked back into the living room.

"Could I take this?" she asked. She didn't know it was a gift to me from my girlfriend.

"Tammy, that was given to me by Betty." Then they selected from Mark's collection of duck decoys on the dining room hutch.

I walked them to the front door to say goodbye. It was all I could do, not to cry and scream after Mark's daughters walked out with some of his shirts and the decoys in their hands.

This chain of events the day after the service for the death of your husband was inconceivable. It took me several weeks to swallow what happened. His children were entitled to have things, but I wasn't ready to go through it. I didn't mind they took them, but not the morning after the service.

This whole scene helped me to clean things out sooner than I planned. I didn't want to go through the emotions again. I looked at the list of things that went to each family member, a few pieces of artwork in the house, and all the fishing equipment in the garage went to his grandsons. The guns, rifles and safe went to his brother. It was overwhelming to look at all the hand and power tools that he didn't mention, and the prints stacked on the shelves.

A few days later, I sifted through things in the house, mainly Mark's clothing and shoes. During his illness, Mark's sizes varied by weight gain. I wanted his nephews or his brother to have whatever they wanted, so I divided the pants and shirts according to sizes. I kept some of his shirts and sweaters for myself to smell his scent. I called Robert.

SECTION 5 - AFTER

"Hey, you think we can transport all the stuff going to Mark's kids to your house? Along with your things? I just can't go through the emotions again, having them come here."

"Of course. When do you want to do it?" Robert said.

"I'm doing most of it now. I want your kids to have things not named. I'd like Jeff to have all the tools. Unless you want some? I'm giving prints to Roy." I replied

"That's nice, they'll appreciate that," he said.

I went into the garage in the morning to avoid summertime temperatures reaching over 100 degrees. Various guns and rifles secured in the safe, and fishing lures, rods and reels, and ammunition stacked in a metal cabinet. The mounted elk, deer, and fish in the garage looked at me. It took me a few days to part with them. All these items spoke to who he was, what he enjoyed, and how he kept them cleaned and in order. It was his identity.

He had baseball, fishing, straw, and sun-protected hats. I kept his hats with sentimental value, the last hat we purchased on a trip to the coast, and his favorite baseball hat he wore at the very last. This baseball hat had a blue denim bill, a tan cap with the emblem of Denali in bold and a Dall sheep. We bought it while in Denali National Park, Alaska, after we saw the white dots on the hilltop of the Dall sheep from our tour bus. This hat he said he didn't need. He wore every day.

It took a few weeks, but when I finished, I was ready to go out of town and do something for a break. Life called me. I could have stayed inside forever, yet I knew I had to continue to live.

SECTION 5 - AFTER

SECTION 5 - AFTER

Chapter 28: Las Vegas
[OCTOBER 2012]

Everything was as usual. Central California in the fall, eighty-degree temperatures, beautiful weather, but this year in October 2012 miserable without Mark. A cool breeze brushed my face an hour ago. I watched the squirrels jump from branch to branch of the Sequoias and heard the songs of sparrows. A neighbor's breakfast of pancakes and coffee floated in my airspace. As much as I loved the life my husband and I had, a change of scenery and clarity were essential to me. Vital for my well-being.

"Mom."

"That's me. What's up, honey-girl?" I talked on the phone as if I died like the annual plants, dried and withered away. The fall weather started to cool. "Sorry to sound so awful. I do want to talk."

My forty-five-year-old daughter, Ann, hesitated. I heard her soft breath in and out. She worried about me. "Tim and I got an invitation. It's a food show in Vegas," she said. From Fresno, California to Las Vegas, Nevada, an hour flight.

My stomach curled. I wanted her to go. I didn't want her to go. I stared out the kitchen window in Fresno, California, and tried to visualize the sunlight outside, calm, beautiful, heavy, but I came up short. I held myself in a cocoon of inner darkness.

"But, I don't feel right about leaving you," Ann added.

"What? What did you say?"

"I don't want to leave you." She nearly shouted. The words enunciated so I would hear them as she meant them. My daughter and I were close. She wasn't being overly protective, just her usual loving self. I captured her words, the meaning of her invitation, and gripped them hard in my mind. She asked me to go somewhere with her. "Where?" I asked.

I couldn't respond. My big toe suddenly throbbed. I'd rammed it into the back-door slider after I ran inside, and I'd bruised it. My toenail bled and the pain throbbed from my toe to my foot to my leg. It felt like hammers pounded my muscles. Just as quickly the kitchen seemed to spin. I gripped the edge of the kitchen island for support. I couldn't go on like this, losing time, losing touch with the outside world. I sounded like I died too. And I had. I drifted into daydreams.

"You don't have to go," she said.

"That's okay, take me with you." I can't believe I said that. I'm sure I shocked her. Being real and honest, it just came out. Was I ready? Yes, I thought. Then I wondered and asked her, "Do you think it's too soon? What will everyone think?"

"Mom?"

"Yes."

"You've lost yourself."

"I know."

"You're scaring me."

"I know. Let me sleep on it."

Her breath again. Soft, soft. I listened to find mine.

I've said that I don't care what people think. But, deep down, I've tried to do the respectable thing. I always wanted to look at my daughter Ann and in the mirror without shame for my decisions. Probably my Catholic upbringing and guilt.

When troublesome events happened, often wondered, how would I get through it? Or I might have said, "Why me?" With my analytical nature, some would say, I mind-fucked a subject. As things occurred, I've wanted to understand, have logical, yet reasonable solutions for issues. In my way of thinking, scenes in my past should have meaning. As I recount significant memories, most have been good. The bad ones - I wanted to believe prepared me for the future.

Did my memories prepare me for a future alone? What good were memories that burned to false ash without my knowledge or my permission? Memories were tricky. Memories had tricked me, and I was cautious. Did they live, or fade like white noise on a flat-lined monitor?

I kept one memory like sharp, astringent pine and woods cologne that healed and cleansed. I held it close. I slept with my fist in my mouth, fell through the sky as my eyes finally shut from exhaustion, rolling through the hills and mountains toward Yosemite and other adventures the year our courtship began. My thoughts absorbed me? I'm the widow that now gets to be a third wheel at a food show in sin city. How can I do this? Still second-guessing myself.

After I awakened, I turned to my closet for comfort, hoping my usual travel clothes would get me back in the swing. But inside the closet, I didn't recognize the scents. Good scents, like baby powder and dryer sheets but beneath that were stronger ones, the dry, warm smell of pine, the hint of sandalwood and musk, the underlying current of earth and mountains and a rush of clear, fresh air. I clung to my favorite travel shirt, wash and wear, short sleeves, green. The hangar bucked from my own hands gripping it or from wishful thinking. "Please, Mark," I whispered. "Give me a sign." How could I go? How could I possibly go to Vegas?

Inside a foreign feeling bedroom, a spacious master bedroom in a house I'd had to live in by myself, alone like a war survivor, I decided on the trip with my daughter Ann and packed my suitcase. It seemed decadent and wrong, even though it was months since I had been out of the house. I flipped my suitcase on the bed with crashing fury, torn in two about going out into the world like a happy-go-lucky traveler. Just an hour ago, I'd been okay. What changed me? Ann's call. A call to start my life again. Shit.

But in implementation, the suitcase became both friend and foe: Support and suck-hole. Guilt ran up and down my spinal column. Rage was a close second, coursing through my veins like toxic acid. "Well, I'm going," I said to no one. "And no one can stop me." I rushed to put more clothes in the suitcase, and because I feared I'd sit on the floor with utter despair, and never get up again in my lifetime.

Two months after Mark passed, I've opened the closet door, closed it, and opened it again. Enough fretting over what anyone will think. I decided to go on the trip.

"Mom, are you packed?"

"Almost. Not really."

"What's going on?"

What was going on with me? I couldn't figure it out. For the last half hour, I stared at the suitcase, found excuses to dust, cleaned up the house even though it wasn't messy. All I could think about was something entirely dumb when Mark and I sat outside at the patio table. He was always such a jokester. He once told me a family of skunks strolled behind me and not to turn. I didn't believe him and quickly turned like a cop coming. Saw striped black and white furs in their catwalk moved around us. I whipped back, stared at Mark with eyes wide open and sat frozen. Fortunately, they didn't think we were much fun. The family of three skunks walked toward the back of the yard and went about their business.

Normally, I would have lost it, laughing hard. Instead, I sat there, entirely and completely frozen. Frozen, as I talked to Ann, even though I moved around the house and looked good like I was going somewhere.

"Mom, what are you thinking about?"

"Skunks," I said.

My stomach clutched. I wanted to bawl. Somehow, I started in the kitchen when Ann called, and I moved to the bedroom again. I kept her talking. I pulled clothes from hangars and threw them into the suitcase before I figured out another way to put my soul in isolation.

After talking with Ann, I prayed.

"Dear God…could you please just help me here. Even a little."

I looked around my bedroom for a sign. I desperately needed God or Mark to give me a sign.

Something. Anything. "Please give me a sign."

Then I knelt at my bedside, and I said, 'Well okay, not a skunk.' I closed my eyes and thought. I slowly inhaled, then exhaled about ten times. I felt peaceful and calm, like a cloud floating on a sunny day. Enough, to give me a day to ponder it. The next day, I went for a walk, always a better thinker outside.

On my walk, I listened to the birds chirping on one tree, smelled the irrigation of the landscape, and felt the sun on my body. I wanted the same energy of togetherness of the birds who congregated on that one tree. It took me back to my childhood.

* * *

As I kid, I visited my grandparents in Cupertino, California to what I thought was their second home. During the summer, their place was a metal barn with beds, a potbelly stove, and crates used for storage and chairs above the compact dirt floors.

I remembered the smell of the wet irrigation ditches, peach, apricot, prune, and plum orchards when I helped my aunts sort fruit. They wore jean work shirts and scarfs to pull their hair away. Together we worked near a conveyor belt with fruit rolling on the top. My job was to pull the culls out. I asked, "What's a cull?"

"A bruised fruit. But, still good. We don't throw them out," my aunt replied.

"For everything bruised?" I asked

"Yes," my aunt replied.

"Oh."

I never forgot those words. Bruised, but still good, don't throw out. Today, I almost apply it to everything and everyone.

* * *

My Mark. My beautiful Mark was dead. He'd died from Alzheimer's. And I had to keep our memories near and alive where he gave them up, even though I realized he could not have fought harder. Robber! Thief! I wanted to scream at God.

It wasn't fair. "God!" I shouted. My Catholic upbringing wouldn't allow me to disparage God, but I couldn't help myself. I twisted back to the bed and leaned over it, threw my favorite travel shirt like a disease into the suitcase. My hands shook. I wanted to crawl under the bed. But whose bed was it? Was it mine? Was this what Mark suffered for so many years, feeling terribly unbalanced and crushingly disoriented, upended without mercy, and so alone?

SECTION 5 - AFTER

SECTION 5 - AFTER

Chapter 29: Transparent Touches
[2012 - 2013]

Death and how one wants an escort from this life to the afterlife is a personal thing. Mark and I had many conversations about it. We wanted our bodies cremated with our ashes spread in the foothills we loved to hike. I never imagined my body inside a box, and neither could he, both claustrophobic.

* * *

Along with the help of Robert and Fran, we drove to find the spot near a stream and bridge we hiked many times. The day we went to the area, the landscape looked different because of the season, dry with a few pools of water. I walked and looked at the tall mature trees, then I stopped. The leaves on branches alive with movement, filtered in sun highlights, and drew shadows on tree trunks that laid on the floor bed. A constant flow of people hiked, and the hum of conversation ignited the air in this majestic place. I thought he'll never be alone.

"Robert, this spot feels right. What do you think?"

"It's your choice. I agree. Looks like the place." He said.

The drive back, I thought about Mark in that box at home. I imagined Jill and Tammy, Pauline, Robert, Fran, myself, Ann, and her family spreading Mark's ashes.

The next day, I walked up and down the long aisles at the Walmart store. "Where can I find thermoses?" I asked a clerk.

"Ma'am, they're in sporting goods. I'll walk you over," he replied. I bought the six clear, plastic, water bottles. After I got home, I called Robert.

"Robert, I bought some smoke-colored containers. Can you come over and help me divide the ashes?"

"Sure. When do you want to do it?"

"In the next week? Is Tuesday okay?"

"Sure, how's morning? Around ten?" He asked.

SECTION 5 - AFTER

* * *

I hadn't lifted the box since the day I picked up the ashes from the mortuary. I could barely lift it. I couldn't believe his whole body was in that little box, the size of a medium shipping box. I called Robert.

"Robert, I don't know if I'm mentally ready. Does Tuesday still work? I'll call Jill and Tammy to confirm. Can you call Pauline?"

"Yes, it does. I'll call Pauline," he said. I didn't look forward to another emotional day, but I needed closure.

Robert came a few days later. I opened the front door to let him in, and we hugged. We walked into the dining room. I placed the box and the thermoses on the table. We both stared at each other. My heart pounded out of my chest.

"Would you say a prayer?" I asked.

"Lord, we give you thanks for giving us Mark, until the day we see you," Robert said.

Robert untied the remains in the plastic bag inside the box. Without talking, our eyes and hands directed our system. I took the first cap off. Robert poured the soil-colored ashes in, and we heard the sound of crystal hitting the thermos, like sand in an hourglass. We took turns holding, while the other one poured carefully from the plastic bag. Accidentally, some of the ashes fell on the table. My throat watered, and I almost choked. We looked at each other stunned and in shock, not knowing what to do. Using our hands, we pushed his sacred body parts back inside the thermos. My heart pumped faster. It was hard to imagine my husband in all the crystals of bone and ash. Still takes my breath away to know we touched those precious, priceless and cherished, body parts of Mark.

* * *

Two months later in October 2012, the day of the celebration was on our wedding anniversary. I prayed for strength for Mark's daughters. The expressionless look on their faces was like a cloud before a downpour. They both walked, sat on a log, and wept. Painful to think of their dad, my

SECTION 5 - AFTER

husband, lay in that bed of a semi-dry and sparsely wet stream. I walked over to try and comfort them. In the middle of those moments, all of a sudden, their uncle Robert hollered out.

"Look over there," he said. I wasn't sure what direction to look but saw what looked like a beam of light shining on the two tree trunks laid on the bottom of the bed floor. The lights shined and formed the symbol of a tilted cross.

In front of the tree trunks, a buck stared straight at everyone, sat calm and knowing, as though he knew us, as if it were Mark's surrogate, giving us approval of this place.

"There's Dad," Tammy yelled out.

Her dad loved deer and the outdoors. The buck stayed for our celebration. Not frightened and didn't run away. I wondered if God gives freedom to communicate with our loved ones after we leave the physical life? It appeared so to all of us that day, to experience those moments was a gift.

* * *

After my husband passed, I awakened. The familiar tenderness of his body behind me, pressed up against my back with his arms wrapped around me. I felt a tingling jolt and heard a sound, like a metallic echo-vibration. The realization gave me a sense he communicated with me. Overwhelmed with it, I cried. I wanted to go back to sleep and continue the dream. As a teenager, I often dreamed, woke up, and resumed the same vision.

The light from the alarm clock streaked across the wall at 3:00 a.m., the exact time my husband usually awakened to pee. I lay in bed and thought about the coincidence of it all. I felt his energy with me.

* * *

A few months later in 2013, our cleaning lady Nancy started cleaning our bedroom.

"Jean, did you put on perfume?" Her voice always carried loudly.

SECTION 5 - AFTER

"What?" I walked from the kitchen through the hallway then I smelled the cologne right away. The scent of my husband floated in the air. It stood out on the marble counter of the antique wood cabinet, like a trophy. I lifted the coffee-colored glass bottle, topped with a rough-edged gold cap. A pea-size amount of cologne underneath, but no traces of a crack were visible. I stared at her, pursed my lips, and raised my shoulders. She returned the same curious look. We both stood mesmerized at what we thought. I finally broke the silence.

"I think I'll put tissue underneath the cologne." I wondered if it would happen again?

"Good idea," she said.

If I told anyone, would they think I was crazy?

* * *

During the year after his death, I had not seen Mark's daughters. His oldest daughter, Jill, invited me to visit. She had three children, all under five. A two-story home, their main bedroom was downstairs, and the children slept upstairs with monitors. At bedtime, Jill said, "Why don't you take my bedroom? I'll sleep with the kids."

"I don't want to take your bedroom. I'll sleep upstairs. I don't mind." I insisted.

"No, the kids might wake up," Jill said.

That evening, I washed my face and brushed my teeth. Tired after I played with the kids all day, I went to bed, and sure I'd fall asleep fast. The next morning I went into the kitchen and spoke to Jill.

"Did you change your mind and come to sleep in your bedroom?" I asked.

"No, why?" Jill asked.

"I saw an image of a body leave the bed and walk out. I thought it was you," I said as I looked in shock.

"I feel like my dad is here a lot. My sister and I have felt footsteps at night at the foot of the bed. Almost like cat paws," she said.

"I felt the same thing one night. I wondered if that was Mark.

SECTION 5 - AFTER

We both felt sure we received communication from Mark. It gave me comfort to know Mark saw his grandchildren. He looked forward to his daughters giving him grandchildren.

SECTION 5 - AFTER

SECTION 5 - AFTER

Chapter 30: Messages
[JULY - SEPTEMBER 2018]

A few years later in July 2018, slipped into habits that were shards for the taking, I think I made a mistake coming to this writing class in Clovis, California; farm country, hot enough for sizzling sounds on the sidewalk. A fan whooshed back and forth in the small classroom at a local Catholic Church. All hail The Saints, God's most Gracious Advocates.

I was the distant newcomer and sat in a corner where I met two women in a writing group of ten in 2018. The spirited, rosy-cheeked woman with curly hair, I nickname, very accomplished editor. She wrote fiction. She won't read today. The other woman, a good writer, with long hair and soulful green eyes, about my age, wrote nonfiction. I was nervous, rubbed my hands to sandpaper in my lap, dropping pens. The editor challenged that day.

The class began. My writing pages were blank and fluttery in my lap, light for this earth, whittled thin for fractured memories, my needs have teeth.

* * *

On the way to Huntington Lake, CA, you'll pass the turnoff to my home before you approach the rolling swing of the foothills. A dense residential community, green in the winter, yellow in the summer, with a community pool made of overly blue turquoise water in Clovis, referred to as Monopoly homes because the hundreds of same-styled homes could be put on a Monopoly board. A holding place for me, a cookie-cutter section of the world I never envisioned as my future. After Mark's death, I downsized from a gorgeously landscaped home in Fresno to this one in 2014. I moved closer to my daughter to get away from the false belief I could survive memories and the house where my husband died. This twelve-hundred square foot home came with a built-in docking station, speakers, and an alarm system with energy-efficient features. Supposedly fresh as a breeze, and entirely modern. The kitchen with stainless steel conveniences

SECTION 5 - AFTER

opens to the great room and dining area. The king-sized mattress, too big, hides heaps of other books beneath it. All my existing leather sofas and pine dining furniture repositioned into this home, like trying to wear a wedding dress after fifty years, buffers, and angles toward a backdoor escape.

On a burning hot July day, I opened my Honda CRV door and barely touched the steering wheel. Pain shot through my fingers, up into my skull. Tears leaked without permission, salty, sweaty rough. I rushed home from the doctor at noon, about to host the editor and the nonfiction writer from our group. Chocolate chip brownies, my forbidden fruit, our pressing decadence. Even though I didn't cook much in the overly shiny kitchen and never baked, I did that day. Fingers in flour, chocolate, nuts, glass bowl clacked on the countertop. Timer clicked-clicked-clicked as a countdown to dessert or like the first day in school. Adrenaline stung and swirled my gut. I was the new kid at school who tried to make friends. I'm a baby boomer. Feelings are feelings, and mine felt like shit.

We sat on the tubby sofa with binders on our laps. I took a deep breath and reminded myself my words matter. We each read while the ceiling fan circled above us, like an oscillating sprinkler shooting our tears around. Those releases bonded us. Laughter followed then tears as the brownies cooled beyond a new fixation on a canvas of courage.

After I read, a suggestion came to dig deeper to reveal my feelings. I thought opening my Pandora box of narrative and scene description was enough for me to engage.

"Are you pissed at your husband because he passed from Alzheimer's and left you alone?" asked the editor.

"Yes, I guess I am," I said after a long pause. I looked backed and forth at both. My face flushed redder, like a whitewater river that crushed me below a raging undercurrent. I didn't expect to surface.

I never said it out loud before. "After my husband died, everyone else's life went on as usual. I was the one left behind to suffer."

"I didn't see that on your pages. How angry are you?" The editor asked. I looked at her and nothing came out. I realized I was a cheat. I cheated them out of knowing me and how I felt all those years I gave up willingly to take care of his life, even though he left me and could not

SECTION 5 - AFTER

remember my name or his name or our love. A blank canvas, I thought, she's right, I haven't said it.

Yet, it wasn't the end of the story. I didn't care if the presumption was I was crazy; I shared the communication I received from my husband on the other side, through his cologne. Shortly after he died, periodic messages came by air love, my lifeline from him.

"What kind of cologne is it? What's it called?" The editor asked.

I had a mental block. How could I have forgotten?

"Oh, gosh! I can't believe it. It's gone." My head felt heavy, fuzzy and overloaded, buzzed with useless mind chatter and worry. Had I thrown Mark under the bus? He was the love of my life. What was I thinking? How could I hate him? I couldn't wait for them to leave so I could look for his cologne.

I walked them to the front door, poured myself a glass of water. I smelled orange zest and powdered sugar sprinkled on the brownies. I never served them. Right on the counter, they sat, easy five pounds for me, the weight of belonging.

After they left, I tore my house apart. My mind wiped clean, and I sat silently with my eyes closed and said a prayer.

"Dear God, please help me…"

I wouldn't have thrown it out, but where was it? I looked in my bathroom. The central drawer housed deodorant, moisturizers, cleansers, toothpaste, brushes, and floss. In front, a black, mesh makeup bag carried mascara, liner, blush, and eyeshadow. In the rear, a tray held perfumes, and at the back, stood my husband's favorite cologne, Chopard, in a plastic bag with no leakage.

* * *

Thinking back to 2012, a few months after Mark's death in Fresno, the cleaning lady started in on our bedroom in our old, shared house, nothing as candy-coated and plastic as the Monopoly home of my future.

It happened; his cologne scent found me seven times in 2013. For some reason, I didn't think to date the scent encounters at first. The last ones were on April 15th, August 23rd, and then on October 13th, three days after my birthday. The sandalwood musk scent floated in the air and drifted from the marble table through the airspace to me. I kept all the aromatic tissues tucked in a copper potpourri on my desk.

Mark's death followed me on a canvas of scent I did not work over with new brush strokes or master with trembling hands. On an artist's sundial of lost causes, this would mean we are all unfinished, forgotten outlines, our souls to the wind. Perhaps on the other side, we are whole, diluted to a pure scent, formed into molecules. When I caught a whiff of his cologne, it was my safe space, a vault.

Not revealed like my anger and emotions.

* * *

September 2018, I took my last trip to the foothills. Evidence of the fires with some charred trees made it look like a war zone. Closer to our favorite area, lovely green sequoia trees, and a hint of fall colors with rust and amber, laced the oak and pine trees to save the day. Near the bridge, areas of trees looked similar, so I compared the photos I had taken previously. Different times of the year, water flowed in the stream near the bridge, called our sacred spot. That day additional fallen tree trunks lay on the dry bed like dead soldiers.

Absence of the bubbling stream's sound, to the twitter of birds, and the flutter of the butterflies gave it life again. The plentiful monarch butterflies lay on the white and grey boulders, which provided a contrast of black and orange color, that I had never seen in this area.

SECTION 5 - AFTER

A Monarch butterfly transforms from one state to another. It starts as larva, wraps itself in a cocoon, and eventually breaks free as a beautiful butterfly. Some believe these creatures are known as symbols and messengers of the spiritual and angelic world. I think the Monarch butterflies were a sign; the adversity I experienced prepared me for the beauty. At first, startled with all these events, I didn't know what to do with it all, but now I'm convinced these messages were gifts from God to let me know Mark arrived. Can I move-on in my journey without Mark?

SECTION 5 - AFTER

Epilogue

I had no idea that Dementia can be a warning sign of many other diseases. It's a gradual precursor that creeped out, and I didn't notice it at first. It played out in my husband's subtle forgetfulness and confusion.

He was ashamed of it, and he didn't want me to tell anyone. I kept his secret. I was in denial of it at first, but the actions didn't go unnoticed by others. I should have told the family members and our friends sooner.

I advise anyone observing changes in their loved ones to seek support early on through local resources. I reached out to the local Valley Caregivers Resource Center, which offered educational classes on many diseases and UCSF Alzheimer's Association, which was specific to my husband's illness and provided crucial support and insight into what we would be facing. Both of these agencies were free when I used them and were a great resource.

I learned so much along the way on this journey. I caution to anyone who is entering a second or third marriage with separate assets, how important it is to prepare ahead of time. Especially, as it relates specifically to health care for an ill spouse, the necessary consideration for the caregiver spouse financially, should they chose to quit work before retirement. The only available government programs for caregiver spouse income are for low-income individuals.

Enormous underlying take away is this - some people marry for financial reasons, instead of for love. No one could sustain the energy to go through this journey unless you married for love.

References

Medi-Cal benefits had the following guidelines: The California Medical Assistance Program is California's Medicaid program serving low-income individuals, including families, seniors, persons with disabilities, children in foster care, pregnant women, and childless adults with incomes below 138% of the federal poverty level.

If more privacy is needed for the sick spouse, it cost other families or the able-bodied spouse a median cost of $7,450 for a semi-private room and $8,669 for a private room in California, by a study of 2015 from skillednursingfacilities.org quoted on 9/18.

Acknowledgments

I thank God for giving me the ability, strength, and courage to write this book. I would not have been able to do any of this without the support and love given to me by my daughter, Ann, her husband, Tim, and my grandchildren, especially for reading the early drafts. Thanks to the many good friends who read the early drafts.

I sincerely appreciate the many writers and editors in my writing circle who gave me feedback. Thanks to my coach, Albert Flynn DeSilver, for his initial guidance and direction, and to Rachel Howard, who edited the first draft. Thanks to my former participants of the California State University of Fresno Summer Arts Program, led by Steven Church and to associate participants of the Clovis Writing Workshop, led by Janice Stevens, and to CJ Collins, my editor.

Special thanks to Gar Reyna, the graphic designer, who designed the book and cover design concepts.

I hope this book helps individuals faced with similar adversities, and to bring more awareness to those who haven't faced it. As well, to help assisted living institutions and hospitals to educate their staff on how to treat Alzheimer's patients or any patient with special illness needs.

About the Author

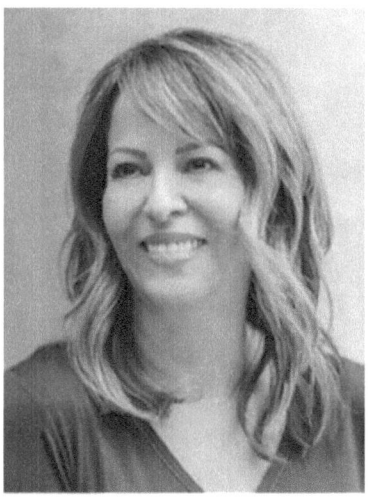

Felicity Jean is a mother, grandmother, seasoned business professional, and currently licensed as a real estate broker in the state of California. She has been licensed as a California Certified General Appraiser, nationally as a Financial Advisor with the Securities Exchange Board in California and Nevada, in bank management, and a graduate of Omega Business School in Advanced Credit Analysis. She received her Creative Writing Certificate at California State University, Fresno, and was selected to participate in their 2018 Summer Arts Non-fiction and Publishing program, and to serve on the Fresno community board of the Summer Arts California State University Foundation.

This debut memoir shares the adventure and fun before her husband's diagnosis, the struggles they experienced, and the gifts she received from him after his death. She wants to bring awareness to this disease that ravages individuals in their middle age and that early financial planning is paramount, especially for second marriages.

Contact her at: FelicityJeanAuthor.com

www.ingramcontent.com/pod-product-compliance
Lightning Source LLC
Chambersburg PA
CBHW021057080526
44587CB00010B/275